KETO SLOW COOKER COOKBOOK:

Healthy and Fast Keto Recipes to Burn Fat, Recipes to Reboot Your Metabolism, Low Carb

MARK ARIZONA

TABLE OF CONTENTS

INTRODUCTION

When I first started on the Ketogenic diet, it was so difficult for me because I had no one to hold my hand and guide me. However, for you, my dear reader, you are lucky because I am writing this book to give you a head start; you won't have to go through all the trouble I experienced. You need to know that once you start on this great diet, you will be required to avoid the mouth-watering carbs and stack up enough fats to account for about 75% of your food.

Ask anybody who has lost weight by getting into ketosis, and they will tell you that it's truly worth it. By the time you finish reading this book, you will realize that there are low-carb alternatives to anything you would wish to eat.
This book will inform you about everything you know about the Ketogenic diet.
It is essential to give you a brief overview of what the Ketogenic diet is, even though you will learn in-depth in the book's chapters.

Fat is usually stored because glucose is used as the primary energy source. This is how people add weight. So, if you lower your intake of carbs, the body goes into ketosis and utilizes your stored fat for energy production.

It is important to realize that the Ketogenic diet does not aim to starve calories but carbs. Our bodies develop in a manner that is built in a way that they adapt to whatever they are fed with. If you stuff your body with fats and eliminate carbs, the ketones will be burnt as the primary source of energy.

Many benefits come with the Ketogenic diet. Read on and learn....

Some people follow this diet as a means of losing weight. Because ketosis breaks down fat that is stored within our bodies, some diets' goal is to create this state of metabolism so as to aid in losing weight. Ketosis diets are also known under the name, Ketogenic diets, or low carb diets. The diet can be regarded as a diet with lots of fats, with approximately 75% of calories being derived from fat. On the other hand, about 20% of calories are from proteins and 5% from carbohydrates.

Furthermore, this diet has a positive effect on serious ailments such as cardiovascular disease, diabetes, as well as metabolic syndrome. It also has the ability to improve HDL cholesterol levels better than diets that are moderate in carbohydrates. This diet has also been used to reduce seizures in children suffering from epilepsy who do not respond to other treatments. However, this is done under medical supervision.

In patients suffering from type 2 diabetes, this diet can be recommended. This is because, with this type of diabetes, the body still produces some insulin but is not able to sufficiently use the insulin in the transportation of glucose into the cells to be used as fuel. The ketogenic diet is focused on reducing the intake of dietary carbohydrates.

People suffering from diabetes who follow this diet need to carefully monitor their ketone levels.

CHAPTER 1: HIGH PROTEIN AND HIGH FAT DIETS

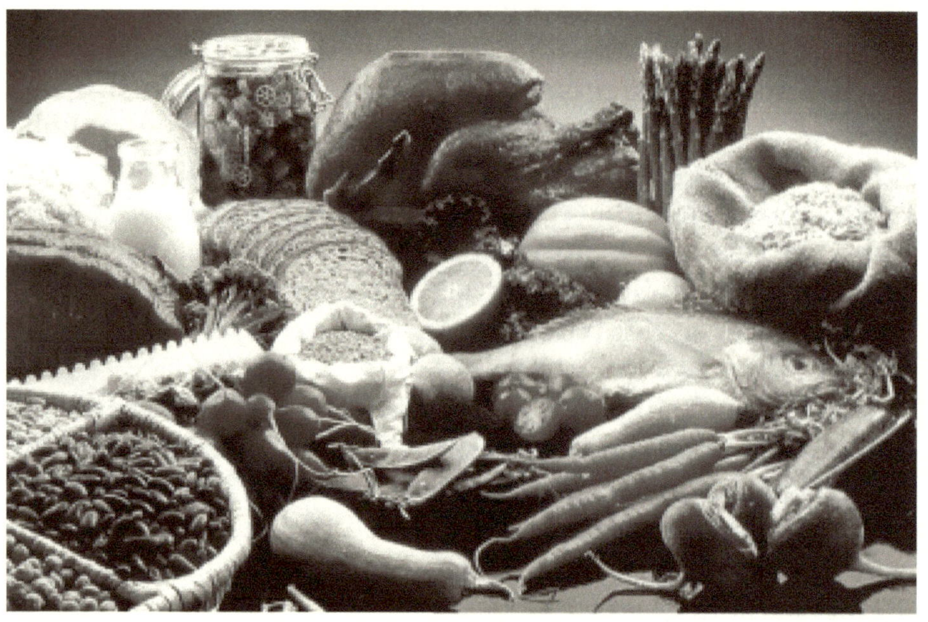

UNDERSTANDING OBESITY IN THE UNITED STATES

There is sufficient scientific evidence to suggest that the two leading causes of the rise in obesity, particularly in the United States, it is widely attributed to overeating food and too little exercise. However, there is a lack of conclusive evidence of the same.

Obesity is a worrying health issue in America. Obesity causes many illnesses and puts sufferers at risk of developing cancer, strokes, and diabetes, among other conditions. Obesity rates have been soaring to alarming rates within the United States, with two in every three people being obese. Obesity also puts a strain on the sufferers' finances. An obese person in the United States spends an average of one thousand dollars more on medication every year.

Furthermore, obesity is one of the contributing factors in the majority of deaths within the United States. The issue of obesity doesn't discriminate, and it has affected all population groups within America for many years. Additionally, obesity has also increased in kids and teenagers. Their babies, on the other hand, stand a risk of being born prematurely, having deformities, and having perinatal deaths.

Obese women are also not likely to breastfeed, and even if they do, they are likely to stop it sooner as compared to healthy mothers. Obesity is, even more, torturing for children and teenagers because they undergo psychological problems due to social discrimination by their peers, sinking them deeper into stress-related eating. This kind of stress impacts negatively on a child's school performance and self-esteem.

Some of the facts about obesity in the United States are:
- More than ⅓ of adults in America suffer from obesity.
- One in every six kids suffers from obesity.
- Over sixty chronic illnesses are linked to obesity.
- Overweight kids have a higher chance of remaining the same when they are adults.
- The larger the size of your waist, the higher the chances of developing diabetes.
- Obesity results in more deaths as compared to being underweight.
- The southern part of the United States has the highest rates of obesity.

THE HYPE AROUND HIGH-PROTEIN AND HIGH-FAT DIETS

In the early 1960s, the ideas of heart Dr. Robert Atkins emerged, and he challenged what people thought was a healthy diet. In short, Dr. Atkins encouraged people to consume meals that had high fat and protein content. This was contrary to what many believed promoted good heart health.

Dr. Atkins was faced with the task of making his case and proving the health benefits of what would become a new diet focus into the 20th century and change the way people thought about food for decades to come. Traditional wisdom put forward the notion that losing weight was a simple matter of eating less.

This belief was the basis for what was then believed to be a balanced nutritional diet combined with foods that were controlled by calories alone. Thus, all weight loss programs were summarized in the notion that if your output of energy exceeded your intake (total amount of calories consumed) over a period, you would lose weight. Enter Atkins with a whole new way of thinking: change what you eat, rather than how much you eat and set aside calorie counting.

This was a revolutionary way of thinking, and some desperately obese and cosmetically uncomfortable candidates were willing to give it a try. They came back with outstanding results—losing significant amounts of weight and enjoying a fitter and healthier lifestyle.

Even today, celebrities such as Kim Kardashian attribute their weight loss to the principles of the Atkins diet. In addition to weight loss, they've enjoyed other health benefits. Today, 'food combining' has hit the spotlight, and conventional wisdom accepts that weight management has more to do with what you eat than how much you put in your mouth.

Thick steaks with a broad rim of fat and topped with cream, were some of the images Atkins used to both shock and delight people who wanted to find out more about this unconventional heart doctor's diet plan. The disbelief was enough of an incentive, and people flocked to meet with him to get the eating plan.

In essence, what Atkins promised was a way to satisfy your appetite, have more energy, and increase your metabolic rate and store less fat. However, it was not only the success of thousands of consumers that brought Atkin's new following. Subsequently, several individuals who followed this diet reported feeling less hungry, more satisfaction, and more energy to conduct their day-to-day activities.

In 1963 Robert C. Atkins sought to consolidate his findings and wrote a series of articles to explain how important it was to control the intake of carbohydrates.

Two decades later, the low-carb diet had become the new normal. Most Americans were eating a reduced number of carbohydrates and not only losing weight but feeling much healthier too. Low carb thinking was soon to blast through consumer consciousness. Soon other doctors and scientists entered the fray with their versions of the low carb diet.

THE ATKINS CAN BE DIVIDED INTO FOUR STAGES OR PHASES

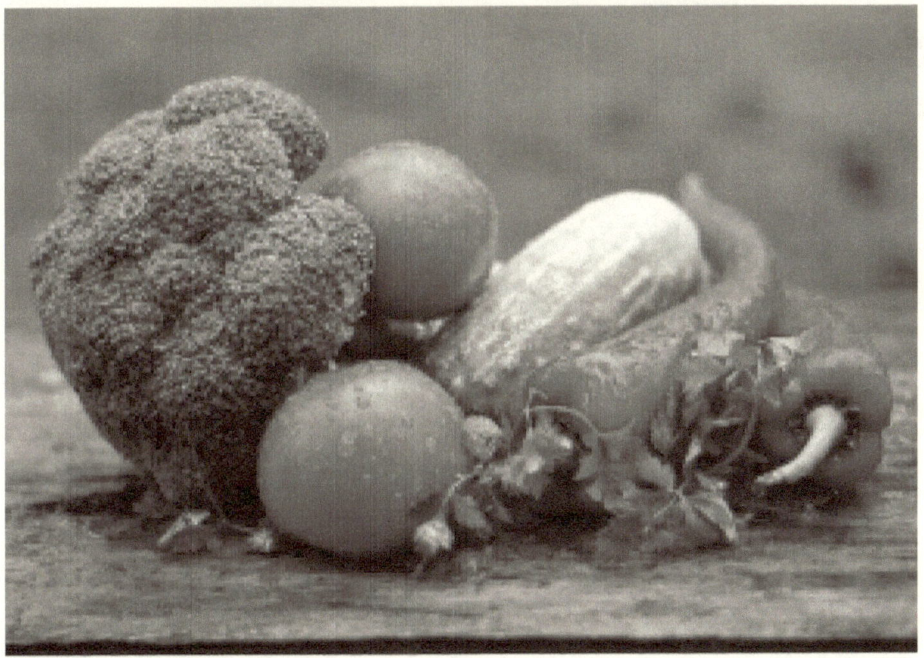

They are:

Stage 1 – This is the induction phase where a person consumes less than 20 grams of carbs on a daily basis for fourteen days. You need to eat foods with high fat, high protein, and low-carb veggies.

Stage 2 – This is the balancing phase, where you gradually include more nuts.

Stage 3 – You add more carbs to your diet up to a point where the loss of weight decreases.

Stage 4 – This is the maintenance phase where you are allowed to eat any healthy carbs without adding on weight.

There are also foods to avoid while on the Atkins diet, and they include:

- Sugars found in fruit juices, soft drinks, ice-cream, sweets, and cakes.
- Grains such as wheat, barley, and rye.
- Veggie oils.
- Trans Fats.
- High carb veggies such as carrots while at the induction stage.
- High carb fruits such as apples, bananas, and pears while also at the induction phase.

Recommended foods are:

- Meats: pork, lamb, beef, and bacon.
- Fatty fish and seafood such as salmon and sardines.
- Eggs
- Low-carb veggies which are spinach, broccoli, and kale.
- Full-fat dairy.
- Nuts and seeds
- Healthy fats like avocado oil and coconut oil.
- Beverages that are allowed on the Atkins diet are water, coffee, and green tea. You can take moderate amounts of alcohol.
- Just know that if you revert to eating the old food in the same portions as before, you will add weight again. This applies to all kinds of weight loss diet plans.

A SEVEN-DAY ATKINS MENU SAMPLE

Day One
Breakfast – eggs, and veggies fried using coconut oil
Lunch – chicken salad with olive oil with nuts
Dinner – steak and vegetables

Day Two
Breakfast – eggs and bacon
Lunch – chicken and vegetable leftovers from the previous night
Dinner – cheeseburger without the bun, veggies, and butter

Day Three
Breakfast – omelet and vegetables fried in butter
Lunch – shrimp salad with olive oil
Dinner – stir fry ground beef with vegetables

Day Four
Breakfast – eggs with vegetables cooked in coconut oil
Lunch – Leftover stir-fry from the previous night
Dinner – salmon with butter and veggies

Day Five
Breakfast – eggs and bacon
Lunch – chicken salad with olive oil and nuts
Dinner – meatballs with vegetables

Day Six
Breakfast – omelet with vegetables fried in butter

Lunch – Leftover meatballs from the previous meal
Dinner – pork chops with veggies

Day Seven
Breakfast – eggs and bacon
Lunch – leftover pork chops from the last meal
Dinner – Grilled chicken wings, salsa, and vegetables

Blending a variety of plants within your meal plan is essential.

COMPARISON BETWEEN THE ATKINS AND KETO DIET PLANS

They both advocate for a reduction in the intake of carbs, but they are different concerning difficulty, results, and safety. In case there was a rating, these two diet plans would be neck to neck because they follow the same principle of low carbs. It is not just about limiting the carbs but even some selected fruits and vegetables. Ketosis is involved in both the diets but in different ways. What this means is that it affects how each of the diets is sustainable in the long term.

Similarities Between the Two Diet Plans
If you follow them correctly, they will both make you lose weight. While on these diets, you are not obligated to count your calories. However, you are required to track the number of carbs you consume.

Differences Between the Two Diet Plans
The first major difference is the amount of protein you are permitted to consume. There is no limit when it comes to the Atkins diet, but the Keto diet limits the amount of protein to about 20% of one's day to day calorie intake.

Secondly, the Keto diet concentrates on the body being in ketosis for the entire period. One is on the menu while on Atkins, ketosis is essential only during the first stage, and probably the second.
On the Atkins diet, you eventually consume carbs, but on the Keto, they are forever limited.

From the above comparison, it is clear that the Atkins is easily sustainable in the long term because it is not as restrictive as the Keto diet.

Additionally, on the Atkins, you can reintroduce nutritious foods such as oatmeal and fruits. However, in my opinion, the Atkins can easily make you add more weight once you reintroduce carbs, unlike in the Keto, where you should always be in ketosis.

Most dieticians recommend long-term, healthy lifestyle changes rather than a rigorous fad diet where weight loss may be quick but unsustainable at the same time. This is conventional wisdom, and people choose what ultimately works for them. The ketogenic diet will produce results, and you will benefit from it in many more areas of health, including mental clarity and focus.

Extreme low-calorie diets make it easier to regain weight after a portion of food is over. If someone with a slowed metabolism hits their target weight and celebrates by eating the same number of daily calories a person with a typical resting metabolic rate or RMR and of their same weight and age would eat, they could gain weight rapidly.

"If you are significantly restricting your calories in the short term, you are going to dampen your resting metabolic rate, but studies show that once you stop restricting food, your RMR will return to the expected for your body weight," Lara Dugas told Healthline. This means most people who diet regularly don't face any metabolic damage. Lara Dugas, Ph.D., MPH, received her doctorate in Exercise Physiology from the University of Cape Town, South Africa, in 2004. In 2007 she joined Loyola University Chicago as a research associate, utilizing her training in the measurement of human metabolism, including whole-body energy expenditure, diet, and physical activity monitoring.

In a study of postmenopausal women with a history of chronic dieting, researchers concluded the same thing: Yo-yo dieting doesn't hurt weight loss or cause permanent damage the metabolism. Also, a damaged metabolism may not be a problem when a person regains weight. People often feel like their body fights to maintain a certain set weight, and this is precise, what's being done!
Pick a diet that you can stick to and "aim for no more than one to two pounds of weight loss a week." When you drastically change the conditions in your body, it can shock your metabolism or mood, he explained.

In local bookshops or even online, there are hundreds, if not thousands of different diets and meal plans that you can embark on.

You may decide to follow a diet because someone recommends it, or maybe you saw a convincing testimonial. You may fail to realize the changes you expected, but interestingly enough, it may work for somebody else. Getting into a diet just because it works for someone else is quite dangerous, and you can even become sicker than you initially were. For example, in a research study that was done among 800 people in Israel, there was a lady that repeatedly had a rise in her blood sugar each time she ate tomatoes. According to the researcher, Eran Segal of the Weizmann Institute of Science in Israel, they were shocked at the considerable variability in how people reacted to the same meals. Subjects in this study had blood sugar monitors that recorded every five minutes for seven days.

The group also provided samples of their stool so that their gut microbiome could be examined. They also kept an orderly record of whatever they ate. No member of the group had diabetes even though some were overweight and were in a condition referred to as pre-diabetes. The researchers were astonished to see a disparity in people's metabolic reactions to similar foods. For example, the blood sugar of some participants rose higher after eating sushi as compared than when they had ice cream.

CHAPTER SUMMARY

- Obesity is a worrying health issue in America. Obesity causes many illnesses and puts sufferers at risk of developing cancer, strokes, and diabetes, among other conditions.
- The differences and similarities between Atkins diet and Keto diet plans

CHAPTER 2: KETOGENIC DIET DEMYSTIFIED

It controls the intake of carbohydrates to a low grammage, only 20 to 40 grams per day for adults. As you will derive a high percentage of your calories from fat, it forces your body to find its energy source here. Instead of your body utilizing energy generated from carbohydrates, it will draw strength from the body's supply of fat. When your body uses energy from fat sources, it enters a state of ketosis.

Eating fat to lose weight sounds counterintuitive and goes against everything you've ever believed about dieting, but fat is essential to support many of the body's systems, including digestive, respiratory, and endocrine. Eating fat is not only imperative for weight-loss, but it's also the key to a surprising number of additional health benefits.

For years I was a sugar addict, starting the day with a biscuit to accompany my sugared coffee, sweetened low-fat yogurt, and cereal for breakfast and more sugared coffee to wash it all down. My lunch comprised a few slices of bread or a nice serving of pasta with a sauce and little protein and vegetables. Dinner was a repeat of lunch with a few pieces of chicken or pork with deep-fried potatoes and more bread. I would follow this by a serving of three scoops of ice-cream or custard to satisfy my sweet tooth after the meal.

No wonder I was ballooning into a state of obesity and ill-health!

Turns out, fat, yes, fat—is your friend. However, before you jump from the fat into the frying pan, know one thing for sure. Fries are out, and not all fats are right for you.

Your body requires healthy dietary fats (such as avocados, omega-3s, nuts, and seeds). These healthy fats provide a variety of benefits that include boosting energy levels, curbing cravings, and lowering "bad" cholesterol. Healthy fats even support your immune system. For years fat was considered a big no-no in any part of a healthy diet, so if you're stuck with disbelief with a different idea about fat, read on.

THE SCIENCE BEHIND THE KETOGENIC DIET

For you to get into ketosis, you will need to make changes and work hard at it even though you will find it more comfortable as compared to other dietary plans since the meal plans will include foods that you enjoy eating.

Start by limiting your carb intake, reaching your day to day macros as well as including MCTs to your meal plans. MCTs enable your body to start the production of ketones, and one should hit ketosis within three days.

You will experience a drop in energy as your body will still be needing carbs; however, within two to three weeks, you will have adapted. If you wish, you can take coffee and other caffeine sources to aid you in staying alert. Furthermore, you may experience flatness and deflation in your muscles due to glycogen loss.

In case you work out since you will be low on energy within the first two to three weeks, you are advised to be reserved and do less of the total sets during your exercise. The process by which your body produces ketones is referred to as ketogenesis. This happens when your body uses fat to generate energy when carbs are low.

THE MYTH OF LOW-FAT

During the 1950s The American Heart Association, US Drug Administration (USDA), and the US Senate discouraged fats due to the risk of heart disease.

For ages, the US media misunderstood 'fat' and reported negatively about it for years. The growing opposition to fat in the human diet began with the rise of heart disease during the 1950s. The total blame was attributed to fat on the menu.

According to an article in Healthline, "By February 1980, the Dietary Guidelines for Americans was issued. The pamphlet recommended against consuming saturated fats, including red meat, full-fat dairy, eggs, and butter".

What followed was a low-fat movement, swapping every full-fat item on grocery shelves for low—or non-fat alternatives. There were low-fat counterparts for everything from butter to cookies. "But these "healthier" options weren't healthy at all. What these products lacked in fat, they made up for in refined sugar and simple carbohydrates. This low-fat crusade did the exact opposite of what was intended: it contributed to widespread obesity".

A recent study examined 135,000 adults in 18 different countries to determine the effects of a low-fat diet. The study found that those who follow low-fat diets consume too many simple carbohydrates and not enough vital nutrients. In fact, according to this research, low-fat diets increase the risk of cardiovascular disease, stroke, and early death.

Healthline adds, "A 2010 review in the American Journal of

Clinical Nutrition showed that saturated fat has no direct link to heart disease, disproving the entire foundation for the first war against fat. Studies like this one suggest that all the things we replaced these fats with—refined sugar, trans fat, and starches—are the real culprits for heart disease."

SUGAR –THE SILENT KILLER

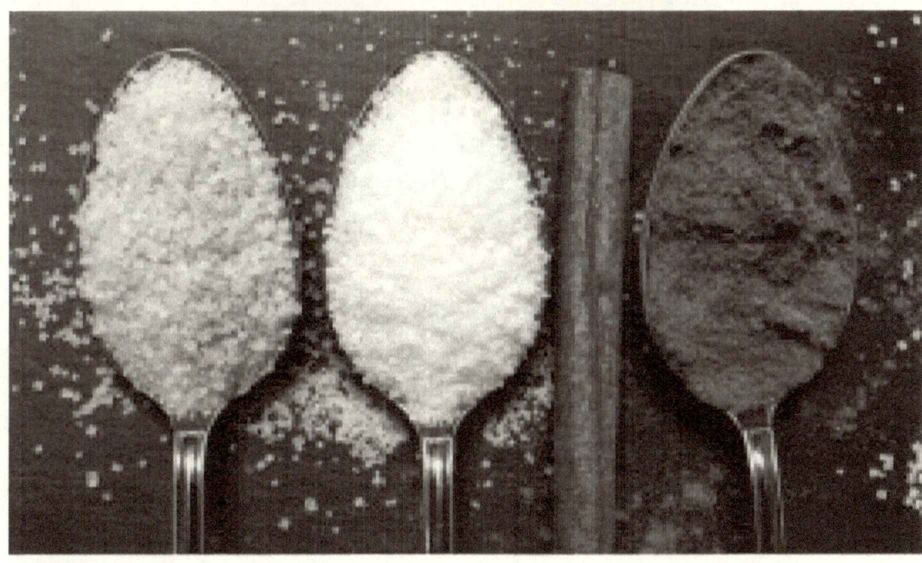

Despite efforts by manufacturers to reduce sugars and produce "light" or "lite" variants in various types of foods, including soft drinks, yogurts, crackers, and even chocolate bars, there is not enough variety of foods and choices available to sustain a healthy diet.

Moreover, sugar is everywhere—it's in your tomato sauce, your mayonnaise, and definitely in your bread and cereals. Even with the most excellent intentions to follow an eating plan, you and the most conscientious dieter will be tripped up by this silent epidemic.

"However, the average Americans are consuming about 22 tsps., or 88 grams of sugar a day, nutritionist Kristin Kirkpatrick of the Wellness Nutrition Services of Cleveland says "we shouldn't be consuming more than 100 calories of sugar a day, but right now we seem to be averaging about 350 to 500 calories from sugar."

A question that often arises is why humans consume so much more sugar than we should? As it turns out, sugar is an addictive substance and has been found to be as addictive as cocaine and heroin.

In a 2007 study, French scientists from the University of Bordeaux allowed lab mice to pick between two types of water; one was water with sugar, and the other was water with cocaine. The mice almost exclusively drank from the sugared water.

Cocaine is highly addictive in mice, and this was the surprising result—it was easy for the scientists to conclude that the sugar was more addictive than cocaine. Dr. Ahmed from Bordeaux explains that this is most likely due to an evolutionary trait, as sugar was almost entirely devoid in human and animal diets up until the recent centuries, which means we consume large amounts whenever it is available, in case the opportunity may not present itself again.

Maguire adds, "the recommendation has now been changed to reduce the intake of free sugars to less than 5% per day, which roughly equates to around six teaspoons. However, for the body to function properly, it only requires the equivalent of 5g (1 tsp.) in the bloodstream at any one time. Why then, do we need to have six teaspoons of added sugar in our diet?"

METABOLISM

Like many aspects of the human body, your metabolism can come from your genetic mapping. This is not the only aspect. Your metabolism will also depend on your weight, age, and lifestyle.

When talking about metabolism, we are referring to the body's rate of efficiency in breaking down energy from food sources. It's always measured at the resting metabolic rate (RMR). In other words, the price will be estimated while the body is still —not influenced by exercise, shock, anxiety, or other exertion.

RESETTING YOUR METABOLISM

Dr. Joe Feuerstein, Director of Integrative Medicine, and family medicine specialist, claims to have found that the ketogenic diet worked well in clinical practice with one patient who lost nearly 100 pounds using this plan. He said the keto diet was very effective in weight loss. Simply put, the keto diet is effective because restricting carbohydrates causes the body to burn energy in stored fat, or ketone bodies. It then breaks these down in a process called ketosis. This forces the body to rely on ketones for energy until you start consuming carbohydrates again.

START WITH SMALL CHANGES

Some carbs are starch dense, like most of the 'whites' such as potatoes, pasta, and bread. Instead, choose carbs that have a much smaller starch component. These include low carb vegetables, leafy veg, and other greens. These vegetables are rich in fiber and will support your digestive system.

Fat is your friend in this diet, but be careful. Restrict your fat intake from animal fat sources. Aim to get most of your fats from whole-food fat sources such as avocados, nuts, and seeds, and olive oil. Variety is the spice of life. Make sure you derive your protein sources from meat, chicken, fish, and dairy to ensure an intake of a variety of vitamins and minerals. Eat fatty fish such as salmon and low-fat meats such as skinless chicken/turkey, loin/tenderloin cuts of beef and pork, and lean or extra lean ground meat (10% fat or less).

EASY WITH EGGS

Eggs are an excellent protein source, but consuming too many egg yolks may increase cholesterol levels. So, you will need to monitor your cholesterol to be on the safe side. Cheese is allowed. You can eat small amounts of cheese and choose somewhat low-fat variants to control the amount of saturated fat intake.

COOKING TIPS

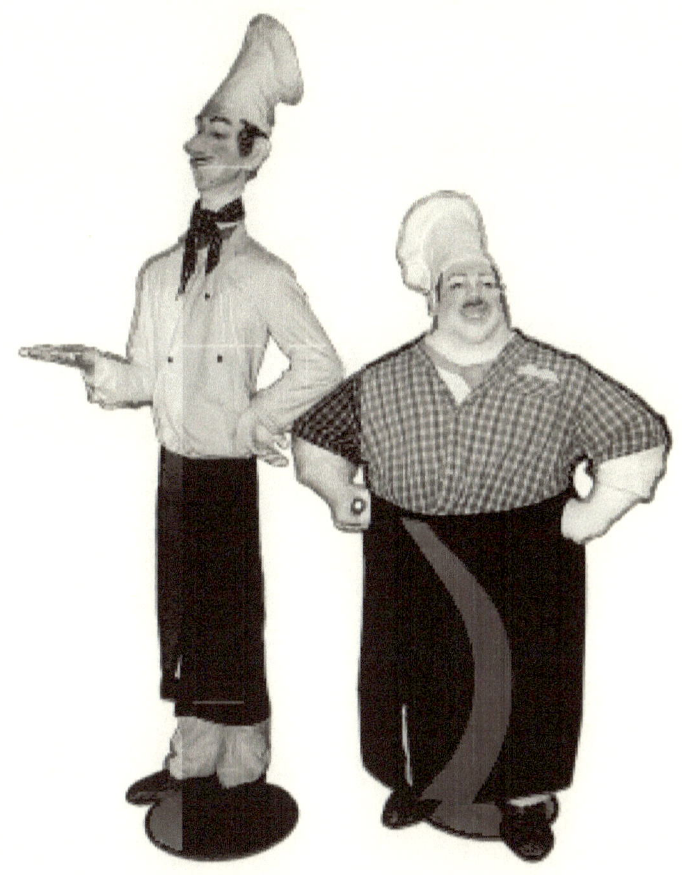

Prepare your food for cooking in liquid fats such as olive oil and other seed oils. This is preferable to cooking in solid fats such as butter or lard. This will also help to control cholesterol.
It's imperative that you allow yourself as much variety as possible from these food groups. This will prevent boredom and help you to get the most nutritional benefit from the foods you

are choosing.

CHAPTER SUMMARY

- After reading this chapter, you have learned
- Ketosis can be achieved by changing your diet
- Why burning fat is more efficient than burning carbs
- Why it is essential to optimize your metabolism
- How to improve your metabolic rate
- Making small changes to your diet can move you towards ketosis
- How to avoid some to the pitfalls

CHAPTER 3: GETTING INTO KETOSIS

Ketosis is a natural metabolic state of the body. This is where the diet gets its name from. During Ketosis, your body will get its fuel from fat cells. Sounds amazing, right? If your body could burn up all that fat for energy, and keep it off your waist? Well, I have some more good news to give to you. That is precisely what it can do.

The entire process of ketosis is started by a tiny molecule in our body called a ketone. They are the lesser-known fuel molecules. While glucose is our body's main molecule for a source of energy, ketones are the only other fuel molecules that can provide our entire body—including our brain—with the energy it needs to function in the same way that glucose does.

Wow, what a mouth full! Basically, our ketone molecules are produced from our fat when there are low amounts of glucose in our system. Our body then burns the fatty ketone molecules up to use for energy.

So, how are ketones made? Simple! The fatty molecules that our body has stored are transported to the liver. Here in the liver, our fat becomes ketone molecules. These ketone molecules enter our bloodstream once they leave the liver and are used by cells in the body for fuel. The exact way that glucose is used.

The reason why ketosis is such a phenomenon is due to the ketone molecule. Unlike most other molecules, the ketone molecule can actually pass into the brain. This is the most important part of the Keto diet! With glucose no longer supplying the body's fuel, your brain needs to get its fuel from somewhere else, and since the brain cannot break down fat for energy, this could be a problem. Luckily, ketones can pass through to the brain and provide it with all the energy it needs in order to help you function. Incredible!

There are two ways to enter the ketosis state, and I will expand on them later on in this guide. Entering the ketosis state can happen through either intermittent fasting or maintaining a ketogenic diet.

Keep in mind that the most amazing part of ketosis is that your brain gets fuel too! And from molecule derived from your fat. Many people assume that the brain relies on carbohydrates for fuel. And while it is true that the brain will consume carbs that we provide it, it will just as happily absorb the ketones our bodies produce as well. That is why eating a low carb diet is essential for the ketogenic diet.

KETO HISTORY

It might surprise you to know that the keto diet was in popular use as early as the 1920s and 1930s. At least this is when it became really popular as an alternative treatment for those who suffered from epilepsy.

The keto diet was introduced as a therapy for those with epilepsy, as studies had shown that previous fasting methods had helped reduce the severity of the condition. As other anticonvulsant therapies (such as new medications) became available, the keto diet was almost all but forgotten about.

Unfortunately, when the medications were unable to help around 30 percent of those that suffered from epilepsy, the ketogenic diet was re-introduced. It is still used as a recommendation today for those with epilepsy—particularly children—as its effects have still proven to be helpful in reducing and managing the seizures caused by epilepsy.

There were many years where doctors were discovering more about the benefits of entering a ketosis state for epilepsy. In fact, the treatment for epilepsy with fasting or a low carb diet dates back to ancient Greek physician's times. However, it was not until 1921 that an endocrinologist named Rollin Woodyat found the three water-soluble compounds in the liver that are known today as ketones. Dr. Rollin Woodyat was able to note that the ketone molecules were being produced by the liver as a result of fasting.

The same year that Woodyat found where the ketone molecules were being made, the diet received its official name from Russel Wilder and the Mayo Clinic before it was commonly used as an epileptic treatment. Shortly after anticonvulsant drugs became popular, doctors no longer received training in the keto diet. This caused a few doctors that tried to use it, to implement it incorrectly. For optimal results with the keto diet, it is crucial to use it appropriately and follow it as needed to trigger the production and release of ketone molecules.

While the ketogenic diet took off in popularity as a therapy for those who suffered from epilepsy, it did not pass by unnoticed the effect it had on weight loss. Even though the keto diet almost disappeared due to a lack of use, around the 1990s, it made a reappearance. It began to grow more in notoriety for weight loss in the early 2000s.

After the 2000s, the keto diet took off in popularity and since then has been successfully used by thousands for weight loss. In recent years the keto diet has taken off due to its advantages in the health field as well. Not only are benefits of the keto diet linked to sustained weight loss and epilepsy, but other medical issues are reported to improve with the use of this diet.

HOW DOES KETOSIS WORK

Now you know how the ketogenic diet came into popularity and the fact that it is achieved by entering into a metabolic state known as ketosis. But how exactly does this work?

When you enter the state of ketosis, you are cutting your body off of its glucose supply. This means that in order to complete those vital life functions like breathing, your body needs to find a different source of fuel.

When you fast or drastically reduce the number of carbs that you eat, you limit the glucose your body can produce. Low levels of glucose send an indicator to the body that it needs to produce energy.

This triggers the body to enter the metabolic state of ketosis. This state can take anywhere from three days to one week in order to obtain. There are a few symptoms you might be feeling during this period, which we will go over later in this guide. Once you are in the ketosis state, your liver transforms your fat cells into the ketone molecules. These ketone molecules are a supplement energy cell to glucose.

Since the keto diet relies on your fat for energy, this is where sustained weight loss comes into play. Because your body and brain will now rely on fat processed through the liver into ketones for energy, it will begin to break down and use the stored fat on your body in the same way. How amazing is that?

The end result, once your body has entered its full metabolic state of ketosis will be a lowered production of glucose and an increase in fat break down. There will be some specific signals that indicate your body has entered ketosis, which we will go over next.

So, how do you know when your body has entered ketosis? It can take anywhere from 3 days to a week (depending on how you ease yourself into the keto diet) in order to achieve the state of ketosis. There are some signs you can look for to help you understand what is going on with your body and where you are in the change from using glucose to ketone molecules for fuel.

One of the first signs that your body is in the full state of ketosis is bad breath. Gross? Well, it is actually more common than you think. Most people report that their breath takes on a fruity smell or a bad smell when they start the keto diet. This is a good sign because it indicates that you have reached the state of ketosis.

The reason that most people on the keto diet experience bad breath is simply because of the compound acetone, which is found in ketone molecules. The acetone is expelled from the body through urine and breath. So, this is why many report that they experience bad breath while on the keto diet.

Most people that are on the keto diet compensate for this by brushing their teeth several times a day and using sugar-free gums or mints. Keep in mind to always check the labels of your gum packets for carbs! You do not want to take your body out of ketosis since you worked so hard to get there.

The other sign—probably the one you will be most excited about—is the weight loss from the keto diet. So, unlike other diets where you lose a lot of weight short-term and struggle with long-term goals, the keto will continue to provide weight loss benefits. This initial weight loss is simply the usage of stored carbs and loss of water weight. After this, your weight loss should be consistent over time, as long as you follow the basic outline of your Keto diet. An effective diet is one that follows the program; otherwise, you will not experience the results you want.

Another marker that you are in ketosis is, of course, an increase in blood ketone levels. There are actually tests that you can buy to test your blood ketone levels! They are the easiest way to test your levels for this sign. This test works by testing for a compound called beta-hydroxybutyrate (BHB) in your blood. The test is a meter that looks for the amount of BHB in levels in your blood. BHB is the primary ketone present in the blood. Remember that a ketone consists of three compounds.

The drawback of testing for ketones this way is that you have to prick your finger with blood, and the tests can be expensive. But there are other signs to know if your body is in ketosis!

Remember that bad breath we spoke about earlier? Well, let us circle back to it. I am sure you have heard of a breathalyzer to test for alcohol limits. I bet you did not know that you can also use the breath analyzer to measure the level of acetone in your breath! And since acetone is one of the three main components of ketone molecules, you will find a good sign about your ketosis state with this method.

The way to find out is by monitoring how much acetone exits your body. During the state of ketosis, your body will expel more acetone levels. While this method is less accurate than the blood meter tests mentioned above, it is still a fairly accurate way to find out if you are in nutritional ketosis.

Nutritional ketosis is just the label for your body's metabolic state of ketosis, where fat is burned instead of sugar.

You can also get urine strips to measure the levels of acetone, leaving your body through your urine. These test strips are a cheaper way to test for acetone levels; however, they are not considered to be very reliable.

For all my late-night munchers and snack fanatics, I have some amazing news for you! Following a strict keto diet has proven to suppress appetites. This is another sign that you are in nutritional ketosis. Decreased hunger is a common symptom of being on the keto diet.

There are still questions in the science community regarding why our bodies experience a decrease in hunger levels while on the keto diet. The main reason we have been given so far is that our body's hunger hormones change with the way we eat on the keto diet. With the increase of vegetables and protein while on the keto diet, the assumption is that these cause the body's hunger hormones to change and impact our snacking habits.

There are some studies right now that also indicates that it is the ketone molecules themselves that impact our brain in order to reduce appetite. So, pay attention to if you feel full and are comfortable, not eating. Especially if you were an avid snack eater before the keto diet, as this could indicate you are in nutritional ketosis.

If your focus and energy increase suddenly, this is another indicator that you are in full ketosis. There are reports that at the very beginning, some people experience flu-like symptoms. This has been aptly named the keto flu. Long-term results indicate that there is an increase in both focus and energy for those that participate in the keto diet.

The reason you might feel sick or sluggish at first is because of the major changes your body is making. You are switching from using sugar as energy to your fat as energy! This requires your body to undergo some changes, and as a result, you might not feel your best in the first week of the keto diet.

But the long-term results and studies all point to significant increases in both focus and energy when following the keto diet. The reason for this is because ketone molecules are a powerful fuel source for the brain. They have even been used in studies regarding concussions and memory loss.

As mentioned above, some people experience tiredness when they start the keto diet. This symptom is only for the short-term, and it, too, is a good sign that you are in the beginning stages of nutritional ketosis.

This symptom is often the hardest for people to manage, and one of the main reasons why they tend to quit the keto diet before realizing its true benefits and rewards. Keep in mind that this is normal to experience. Your body has been used to running on carbohydrates, and the switch to ketones can be taxing on your body.

Prepare yourself for this symptom, and I promise you there is a light at the end of this short-lived tunnel. The best way to prepare for the fatigue experienced during this phase of the switch is to increase your electrolytes. These are best received from supplements that you can drink. A good guide to go by when adding supplements is to try and manage around 1000 mg of potassium, 300 mg of magnesium, and 2000 mg of sodium. This will help your body with the shock of no longer receiving the salt from processed foods.

A short-term performance decrease is another natural symptom. Because of the loss of carbs in your system, you might experience a decrease in your exercise performance. But as with the other short-term symptoms, once your body is used to operating on the ketone molecules, your exercise performance should increase to normal levels.

Allow your body to adjust to the change, and give yourself time to adjust as well.

Because the keto diet involves major changes to the ordinary diet, expect a few digestive issues to follow. Constipation and diarrhea are common during this stage, as they are common symptoms that follow any major dietary shift. Once the transitional changes are over, these symptoms should stop.

In order to ensure that your body's systems remain running as smoothly as possible, be mindful to eat vegetables that contain a lot of fiber.

The final most common symptom that comes from the initial diet change is insomnia. Many people experience some insomnia or waking up in the middle of the night, having difficulty getting back to sleep at night when they switch their diet to the keto diet. This is mainly due to the drastic reduction in carbohydrates.

Once you are adapted to your new keto diet, your sleep should improve in the long-term. With the keto diet, it is important that you note it is not about short-term goals. While there are many health benefits to the keto diet, as I mentioned earlier, this can be a lifestyle change! So, the benefits you are looking at are on a long-term plan.

But these benefits are achievable and within reach of anyone who follows the ketogenic diet.

CHAPTER 4: HOW THE KETO PLAN WORKS

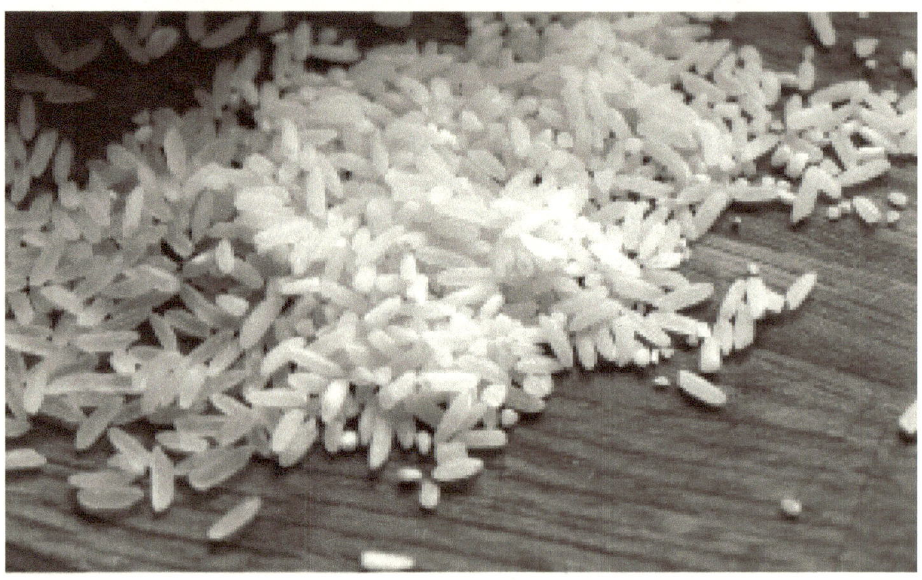

To achieve weight loss, you will need to reduce your carbohydrate intake. Soon, you will realize the plan will allow you to feel full and satisfied while still losing weight. You restrict your carb intake, including starches such as bread and pasta, as well as sugars and replace them with fat and protein. Not only will you lose weight, you will also lower your blood pressure, triglycerides, and blood sugar.

What works for one person as a 'low-carb' diet may be too low for another person. It depends on your activity levels, age, body composition, and gender. It may also depend on your metabolic

health, food culture, and personal preferences.
If you are more active and have more muscle mass, you can tolerate more carbs than someone who is sedentary. If people become affected by metabolic syndrome, they may become obese or suffer from type II diabetes, where the rules change. It is sometimes referred to by scientists as 'carbohydrate intolerance.'

As mentioned, there's no set rule for carb intake. The following are some basic guidelines to consider as you begin the ketogenic diet plan, which is effective about 90% of the time:

MODERATE CARB INTAKE: 100-150 GRAMS DAILY

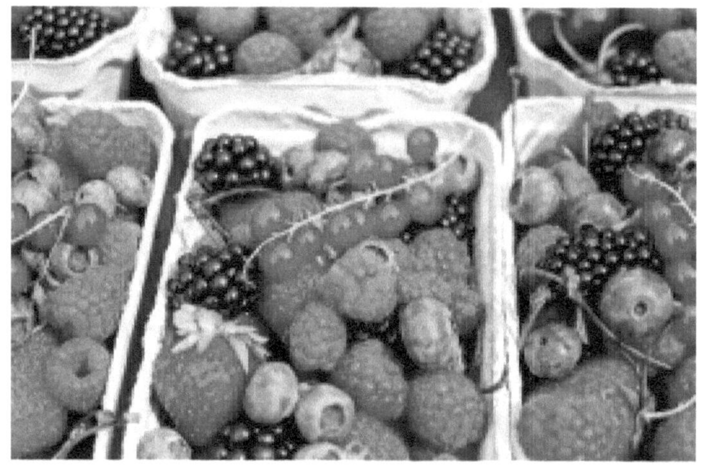

If you are active and lean and just trying to maintain weight, these are some of the foods to consider:

- Several fruits daily
- All the veggies you can eat
- Healthy starches such as rice, oats, sweet potatoes, and potatoes

50-100 Grams Daily

- Plenty of veggies
- 2-3 pieces of fruit each day
- Minimal intake of starchy carbs

20-50 Grams Daily

Losing weight quickly falls into this category. If you have diabetes, are obese, or metabolically deranged, this is the plan for you. Consuming less than the 50 grams daily, your body will achieve a state of ketosis which supplies the 'ketone bodies.' Consider the following guidelines:

- Berries with whipped cream
- Plenty of low-carbohydrate veggies
- Trace carbs from foods including nuts, seeds, and avocados

Before you make any changes, it is important to experiment and categorize where you fall on the scales. Seek your doctor's advice before changing your eating patterns. In some cases, you could reduce the need for some medications.

IS THE KETOGENIC DIET FOR EVERYONE?

The Ketogenic diet or the keto diet is not suitable for everyone. Experts suggest that people with certain medical conditions should not follow the keto diet.

Anyone with one or more of the following medical conditions should not attempt this diet:

- Kidney Failure
- Fat digestion disorders (pancreatitis, gallbladder disease, gastric bypass)
- Genetic metabolic defects
- Beta-oxidation defects
- Fatty acyl dehydrogenase deficiency
- CPT I/II deficiency
- Pregnancy
- Liver functional disorders

GUIDELINES TO TRANSITIONING INTO THE KETO DIET

It is a challenging process to choose to change to a lifestyle with fewer carbohydrates. It takes a lot of willpower to stay away from the tempting treats that your family and friends can consume and not gain an ounce of body fat from. However, you will be ahead of the game plan by using some of the following suggestions. The keto plan works, and you can use it whether you are at home or on-the-go. These are the guidelines:

JOURNALIZE

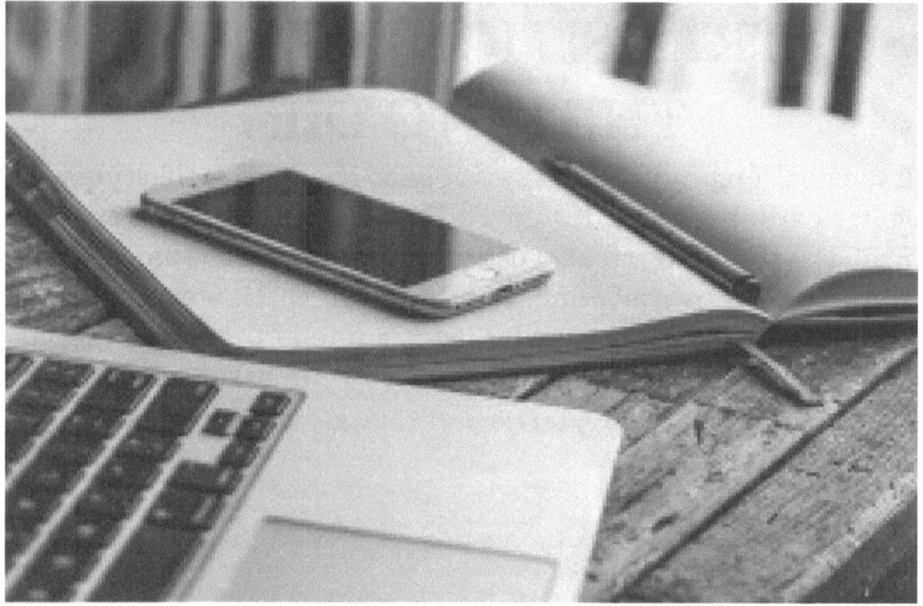

Keep a journal/log of everything you eat. If you cheat, write it down too. It will be a reminder of your indulgence, but it will help keep you in line. Others may believe you are obsessed with the plan, but it is your health and well-being on the line, so don't pay them any mind.

COUNT THE CARBS

Today, almost every consumable product that you buy has nutrition facts on the packaging, so you can keep your carbs in check before you even get home. It might be a difficult process at first, but it is worth the effort. Take a bit of extra time when you plan a shopping adventure.

TAKE CONTROL OF THE KITCHEN

One of the easiest ways to stick to the diet is to remove the temptations. If you live alone, this is an easy task, but it is a bit more challenging if you have a family. The diet would also be good for them if you plan your meals using some of the recipes included in this book. Remove the ready to eat chocolate, candy, bread, pasta, rice, and sugary sodas you have in the kitchen.

STORE TIME

Armed with your new skills, visit the grocery store. Take a well-planned grocery list and read those labels. When you get home, you will feel good to know that you have removed the temptations from the shelves.

BUSY, ON-THE-GO METHODS

If you live a hectic lifestyle, as many individuals and families do in today's fast-paced society; try some of the following recommendations:

EATING-OUT STRATEGIES

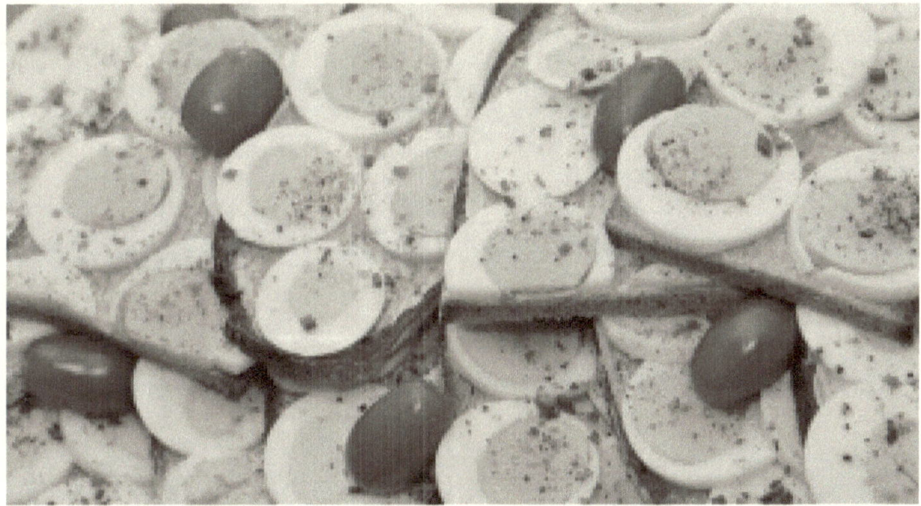

When you choose to dine out, be smart, and do some online research before you leave the house. Many restaurants have an online presence that makes dieting a less daunting adventure. As you continue with your planning, it will become easier, and you can branch out to other locations with the knowledge gained. The following are a few recommendations that might help:

Breakfast: Sometimes, if you want to play it safe, there is nothing better than eggs. You may be off on some of the counts, but after you have used some of the recipes in this book, you will know how to gauge your eating habits for the most important meal of the day.

Lunch: Fish and chicken are usually good choices. Try something like chicken salad or a regular salad. For the dressing, try some vinaigrette or plain vinegar.

Dinner: As your main course, always choose a fresh green veggie with a lean cut of meat. Try something like a hamburger minus the bun, or a tempting entrée of broccoli and steak.

HOW TO FOLLOW THE KETO DIET

By now, you should have a general idea of the concept of a ketogenic diet. You probably want to get started and begin your keto diet immediately, but first, you should clear out all non-ketogenic foods from your pantry or kitchen. Get rid of any unhealthy processed and ready-to-eat foods. Before you go shopping, you can make a list of the foods that are ketogenic and non-ketogenic. It can actually be quite frustrating trying to figure out what you should and should not buy while you are on a diet, so I will help you get started with this.

FOODS TO AVOID

1. Grains in the form of wheat, barley, rye, sorghum, corn, bulgur, oats, quinoa, amaranth, rice, millet, buckwheat, etc. Avoid any bread, pasta, cookies, or even pizza crusts made from these grains. All grains should be avoided on a low carb diet since they will slow down the weight loss process.

2. Beans or legumes in the form of kidney beans, pinto beans, green peas, lima beans, fava beans, black beans, chickpeas, lentils, white beans, cannellini beans, etc. The high starch content in beans makes them unsuitable for a keto diet.

3. Fruits like bananas, oranges, pineapples, papaya, grapes, mangoes, apples, and tangerines. Avoid any fruit syrups, packaged fruit juices, fruit concentrates or even dried fruits. Everyone says fruits are healthy, but they are not keto-friendly, due to their high sugar and carb content.

4. Starchy vegetables like sweet potatoes, peas, yams, corn, yucca, cherry tomatoes, carrots, or parsnips. These vegetables are not suitable for a keto diet as they contain high carbs.

5. Sugar in the form of honey, agave nectar, cane sugar, turbinado sugar, maple syrup, high fructose corn syrup, etc., should be avoided in any form.

6. Milk and low-fat dairy products like shredded cheese,

fat-free butter, low-fat cream cheese, skimmed milk, low fat whipped cream, low-fat yogurt, etc.

7. Factory farmed animal products like grain-fed meats, canned meat, beef jerky, packaged sausages, bacon, chicken nuggets, fish sticks, corned beef, salami, hot dogs, or factory-farmed fish.

8. Unhealthy fats in the form of canola oil, safflower oil, soybean oil, grapeseed oil, sunflower oil, corn oil, or peanut oil.

9. Alcohol like beer, wines, cocktail, and flavored liquors.

10. Sweetened beverages like sodas, diet sodas, juices, tea or coffee with sweeteners, milk products with sweeteners, etc.

11. Packaged cookies and cakes or candies and ice creams. Avoid almond milk products and foods with gelatin.

12. Avoid any artificial sweeteners like Equal, Splenda, Saccharin, Sucralose, etc.

13. Avoid fast food from any restaurant.

14. Don't eat margarine instead of butter, as it is an industrially modified form of butter with too much omega 6 fat and no nutritional benefits.

15. Avoid condiments with any unhealthy oils, added sugars, or low-fat labels.

FOODS TO EAT

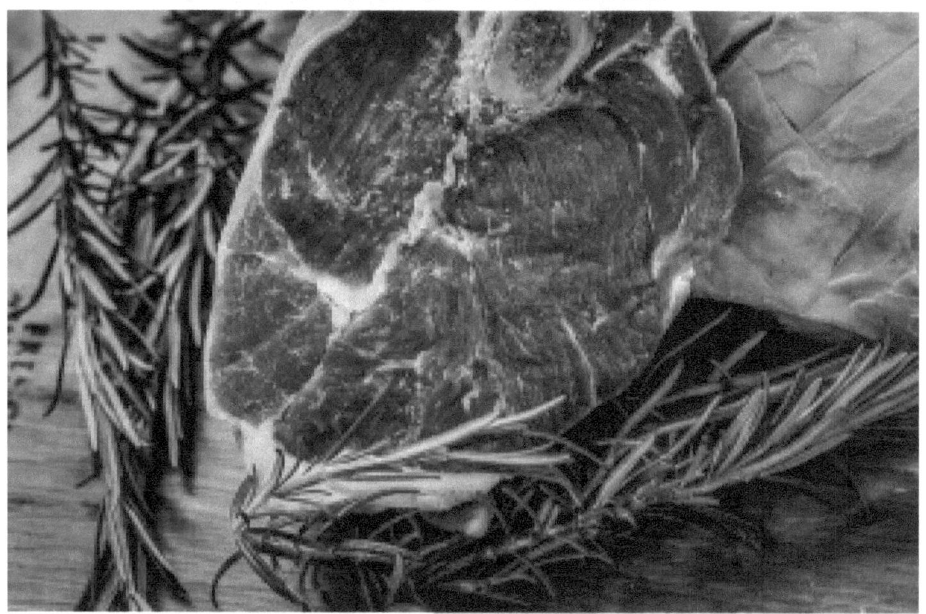

Eating unprocessed meat that is low in carbs is keto-friendly. Any organic or grass-fed meat is usually appropriate for a keto meal. Remember not to overeat on meat as your protein intake has to be moderate, and fat intake increased. If you eat too much meat, you eat too much protein, and this gets converted to glucose for energy.

Fish and seafood are extremely keto-friendly. Try to get fresh and wild fish and avoid eating fish that were bred. Fatty fish like salmon is a great choice.
Eggs cooked in any form are keto-friendly. Try to acquire organic eggs.
Eat vegetables that grow above ground and avoid root vege-

tables like potatoes. Leafy and green vegetables are the best choice. You can also add cauliflower, zucchini, broccoli cabbage, and avocado to your diet. Cook them in fatty butter or oil to make it keto-friendly. Add more vegetables to your plate to make up for the grains you will avoid on keto.

High-fat dairy like butter, cheese, heavy cream, etc. is suitable for a keto diet. The more fat, the better; however, try to avoid milk since milk sugar adds up. Always eat full-fat yogurt and keep away from the low-fat kind.
Nuts are great, but they should be eaten in moderation, as it is easy to overeat on them while snacking. Cashews should be eaten minimally since they contain a lot of carbs.

Low-sugar fruits like berries are keto-friendly in moderate amounts. Berries are a good substitute for sugary desserts. Add some full-fat whipping cream to a bowl of berries for your sweet fix.
Coffee is fine if you don't add any sugar. If you really need to add milk, ensure to use very little full-fat cream milk.
Water is the best liquid to hydrate with. You can add natural flavoring to your water like cucumbers, lemons, etc. to drink more often.
Tea of any kind is healthy, but don't add sugar. On the keto diet, certain teas like green tea or oolong tea actually help to lose weight faster.

Bone broth is highly recommended on a keto diet, as it contains a lot of nutrients and electrolytes and is very simple to prepare. Adding a bit of butter to it makes it taste better and is keto effective as well.
If you want alcohol for a special occasion, try dry wine or any alcohol without sugar, and only have a single glass.

Dark chocolate can be a treat for a cheat day. Buy dark chocolate with high amounts of cocoa, and you can use this to prepare keto desserts as well.

Fats and oils are usually avoided or prohibited on all other diets; however, we encourage you to add these to your keto diet. Fats can be very helpful in losing weight as long as they are the right kind of fats. A keto diet guides you in consuming more healthy fat in your diet every single day. The fats you should avoid are in potato chips, cookies, and other processed snacks. You need more monosaturated fats like those in butter, tuna, avocado, etc. Omega 3 is another nutrient that you need to add to your diet. Fish is the best source for this, but supplements are also available in most stores. Hydrogenated fats should also be removed from your diet. These are usually in the form of vegetable oils. Increase your fatty oil intake with food like chicken fat, beef tallow, olive oil, butter, and avocado.

In a ketogenic diet, proteins are required in a moderate amount. They should be consumed in lower amounts than fat, but more than carbs. Proteins help to prevent hunger and increase energy levels. For protein sources, look for organic and grass-fed options. Eggs are keto-friendly and have lots of protein, but try to buy free-range eggs. Fish, red meat, poultry, and shellfish are also healthy sources of protein.

A lot of people don't enjoy eating vegetables, but you need to remember that they are an essential part of any diet, as they are filled with nutrients that other sources can't always provide you. Those that grow above ground are more keto-friendly than the vegetables that grow below ground. Leafy greens are a very good addition to your diet and actually help you feel full faster. Try to buy fresh vegetables that are organically grown and free from pesticides. If you like gardening, you can go the extra step and grow your own vegetables. This way, you know exactly what goes in your stomach without worrying about chemicals. You can't load up your plate with every vegetable since some are quite high in starch and sugar. The most ketogenic vegetables are celery, asparagus, mushrooms, onions, broccoli, avocado, and romaine lettuce.

When shopping for ketogenic foods, beware of foods that are labeled low carb or keto-friendly. Don't trust commercial products at face value and read the list of ingredients provided on the label. There are always hidden ingredients that you really need to avoid. Packaged foods are usually unhealthy and don't help to lose weight no matter what the label says. These days, there are many products on the shelves labeled low fat, low carb, diet, ketogenic, etc.; however, most of these have hidden ingredients that will harm you in the long run. Any food with artificial sweeteners, additives, alcohol, etc. should be avoided. Remember, you cannot replace real sugar with marketed fake sugar. Also, beware of labels since companies often lie to sell their products.

Raw, full-fat dairy products are also ketogenic. Heavy whipped cream, cheese, sour cream, etc. are all good sources of vitamin D and proteins. They should not be taken in excess but can be added to your diet.

Nuts are a very healthy snack, as long as you can control yourself from eating too much of them. They are packed with protein and nutrients, and a small amount is more than enough. Roasting nuts are a good way to get rid of any pesticides or additives that might be harmful. Amongst nuts, avoid eating too many cashews, and also avoid peanuts as they are a legume and are not ketogenic friendly. If you buy packaged nuts, buy the unsalted variety. Healthy options for nuts include pistachio, walnuts, sunflower seeds, macadamias, and almonds. It is recommended not to have more than a handful of nuts every day, as just a small amount every day will give you a good source of omega 6 and protein.

When following the ketogenic diet, one of the most common symptoms or side effects is dehydration, as this diet has a diuretic effect that can be harmful if you do not hydrate your body sufficiently. This is more prominent in the first few weeks of the keto diet. So, always carry a bottle of water with you during this time, as this will keep your body cool and hydrated. During the first few days, you need to remember to drink twice the amount of water that you usually drink. In the long run, dehydration can have detrimental effects on your body. Aside from water, you can also drink herbal teas, unsweetened tea or coffee, and fruit water.

During a keto diet or any healthy diet, your best bet is to eat real, wholesome food and home-cooked meals. The more minimally processed your ingredients are, the better it is for you. Ideally, buy raw fresh ingredients, and nothing canned or labeled. Also, remember that it is a low carb diet and not a no-carb diet, so you just need to keep the carbs to a minimum every day. The diet does not have to be stressful for you. While following the keto diet, you can eat without staying hungry and still lose weight. If you follow the diet properly, it will have a very beneficial effect on your health and a positive impact on your life, as eating right is extremely important.

The nutritional strategy of a keto diet is to consume high fat, moderate amounts of protein, and minimal carbs. This will help your body enter into a state of ketosis, thereby resulting in the production of the ketone bodies. Your body will soon turn into a fat-burning machine, helping you achieve your goal weight.
Remember, fat is an essential macronutrient that plays a major role in the ketogenic diet, and it is not the fat that actually makes you fat!

SIMPLIFIED LIST OF VEGETABLES TO EAT ON A KETOGENIC DIET

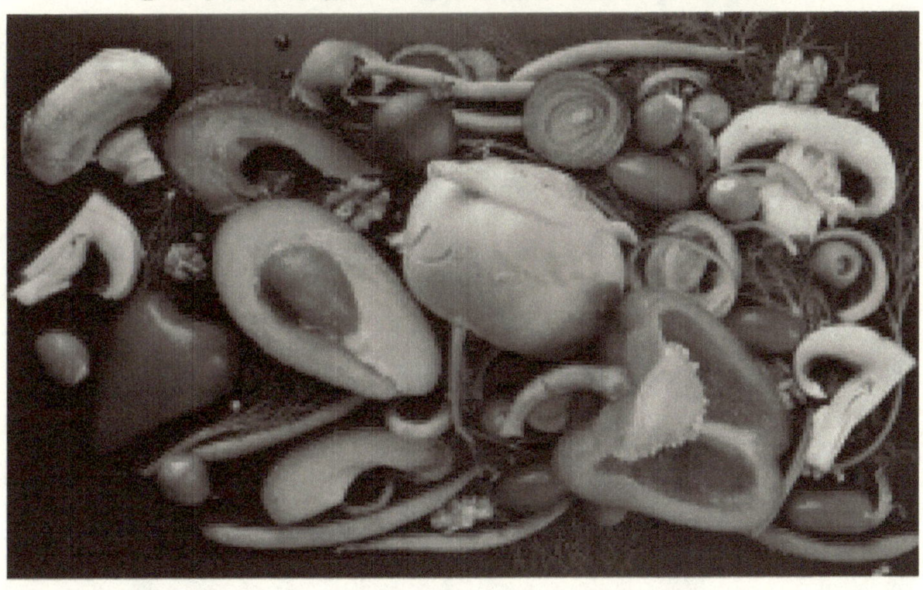

It is important to begin your diet with natural and whole single-ingredient foods. You can include any or all of the following food items to your keto food list.

VEGETABLES THAT GROW ABOVE THE GROUND

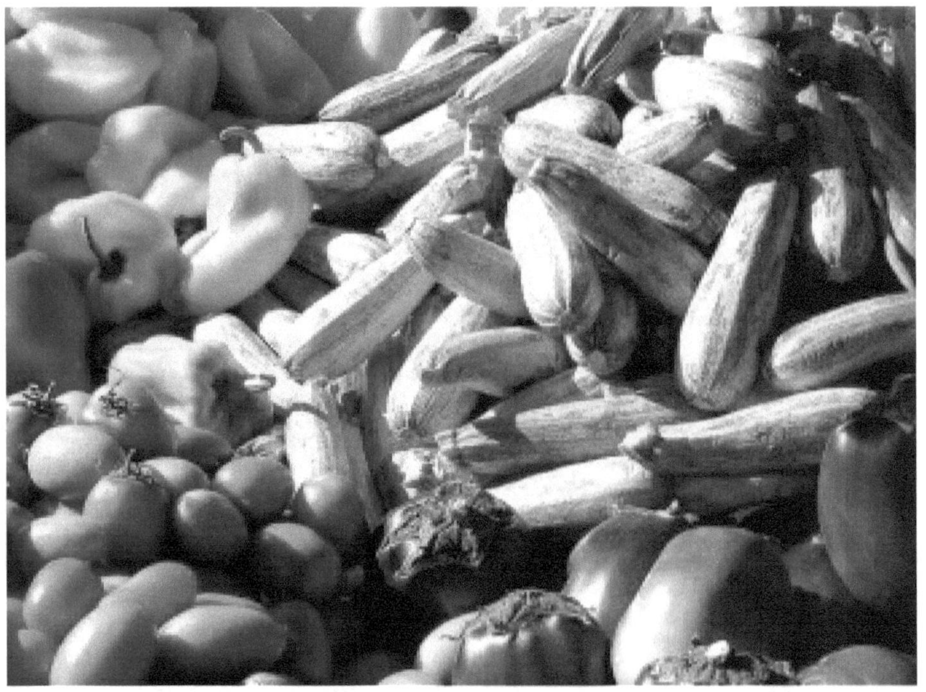

When you include vegetables in your diet recipes, you are free to use either fresh veggies or frozen ones. On a keto diet, the best way to get some good fat into your body is by including vegetables—the ones that grow above ground:

- All leafy green vegetables
- Cauliflower
- Broccoli

- Cabbage
- Zucchini
- Avocado
- Bell peppers
- Mushrooms
- Asparagus
- Peas
- Beans (Green, black)
- Tomatoes
- Lettuce
- Kale
- Cucumber
- Brussel Sprouts
- Celery
- Eggplant
- Artichokes

You can cook the vegetables with olive oil, coconut oil, or butter and allow more healthy fats to get into your system. When you are preparing a vegetable salad, you can use olive oil as your dressing. Veggies are your best fat-delivery system, and they can add more flavor, color, and variety to your keto diet meals.

On a keto diet, you will end up eating more vegetables, as you will need to replace your rice, potatoes, and pasta with mixed vegetables.

OTHER SPICY VEGETABLES

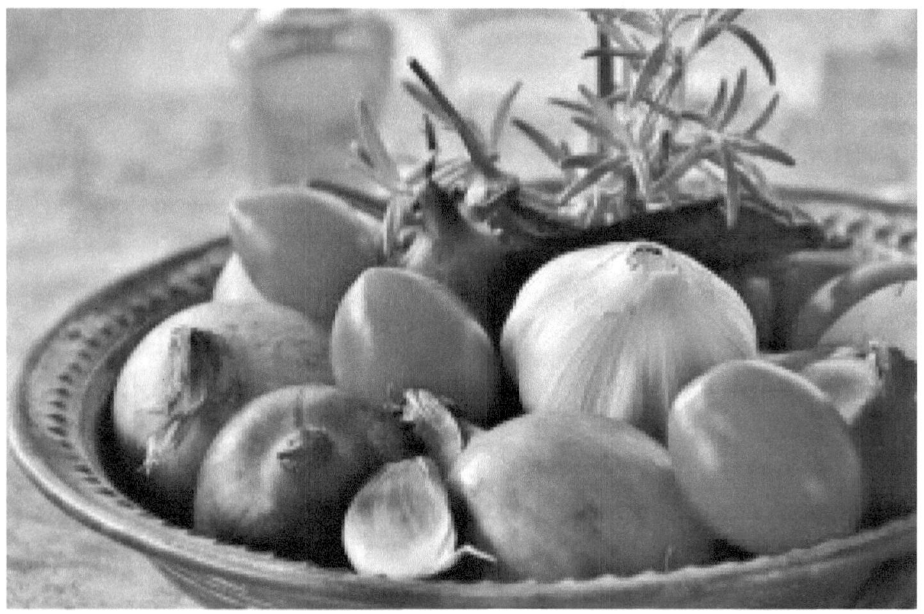

You can also add other veggies, like:
- Onions
- Garlic
- Ginger
- Radish
- Turnip

SIMPLIFIED LIST OF HEALTHY FATS TO INCLUDE IN THE DIET

Avocados, seeds, and nuts are the main food items rich in healthy fats. When you choose nuts, try to avoid cashews, as they are high in carbs.

NUTS

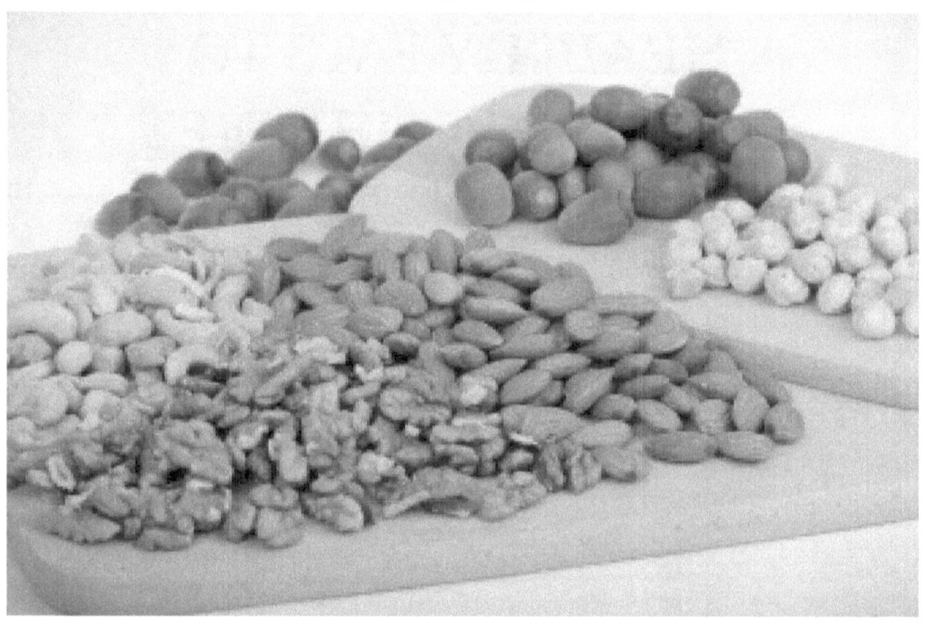

Always go for:
- Pecan nuts
- Macadamia nuts
- Almonds
- Brazil nuts
- Walnuts

Also, you can include nut butter to your food list, but when you are snacking on nuts, you need to be a little careful as you tend to consume more than you need to feel satiated.

SEEDS

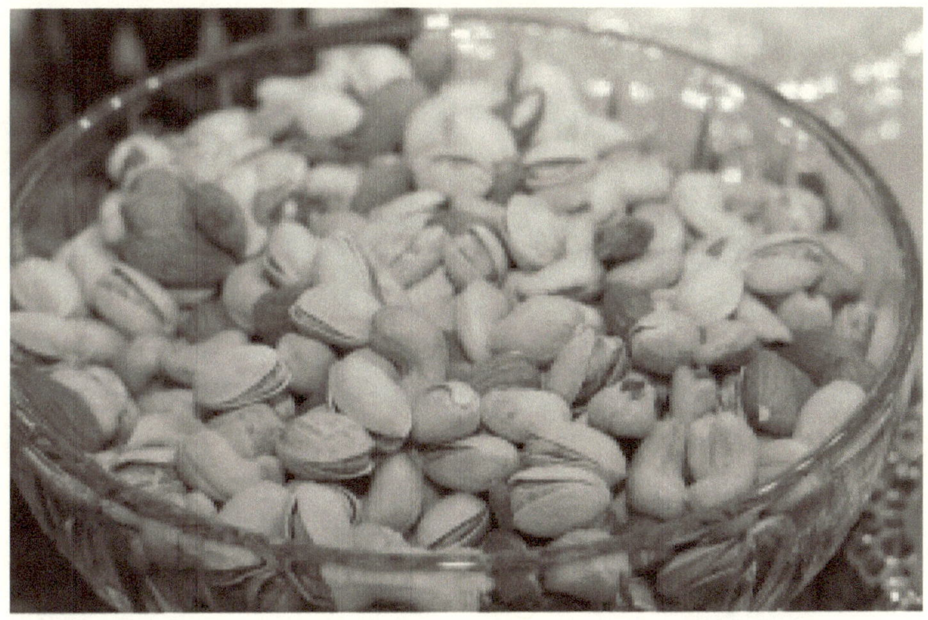

Seeds are also good sources of healthy fats. Include the following seeds in your keto recipes:

- Pumpkin seeds
- Pistachios
- Chia seeds
- Flaxseeds

HEALTHY OILS TO USE

- Coconut oil
- Olive oil
- Avocado oil

SIMPLIFIED LIST OF FRUIT TO INCLUDE IN THE DIET

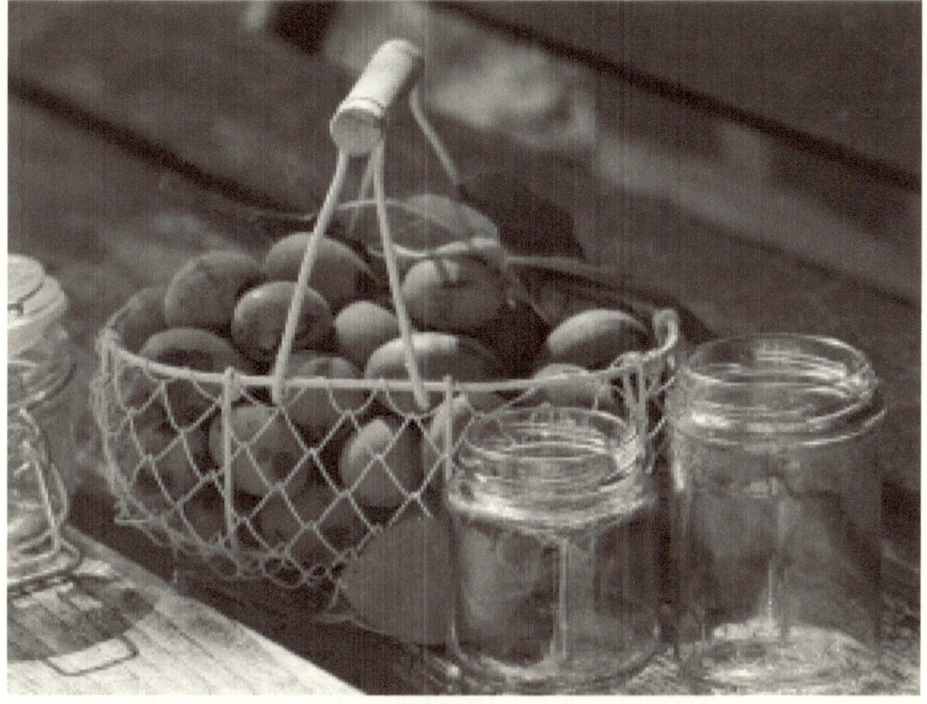

You can include a moderate amount of berries to your keto diet.

- Strawberry
- Blackberry
- Raspberry

Blueberries have more carbs, so be careful when using them, and only use one or two occasionally.

A few other fruits that you can include in your keto diet are:

- Plum
- Cherries
- Peach
- Mandarin
- Cantaloupe
- Kiwi
- Lemon
- Coconut (the white fleshy thing – the meat of the coconut)

SIMPLIFIED LIST OF MEATLESS PROTEINS

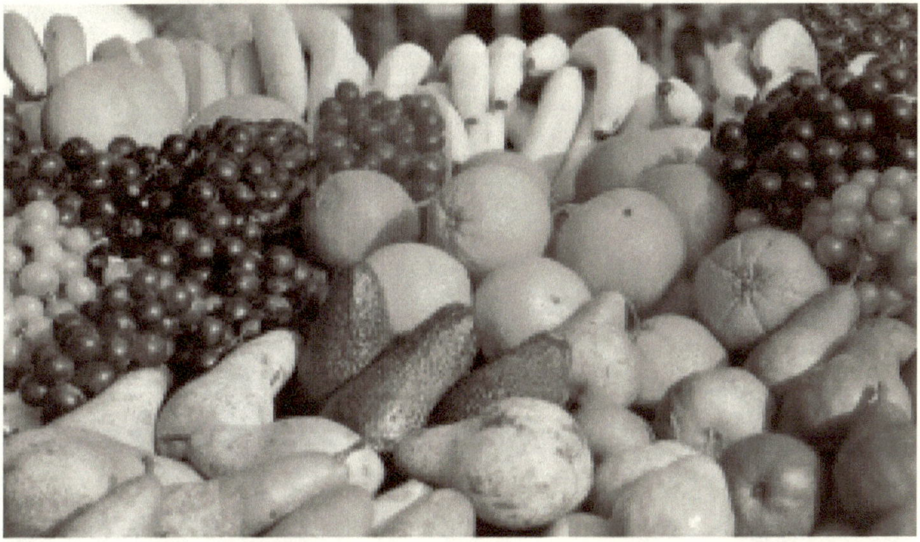

If you are planning on starting a completely vegetarian or vegan keto diet, you can include the following meatless options:

- Seitan
- Tempeh
- Tofu

CONDIMENTS TO USE ON A KETO DIET

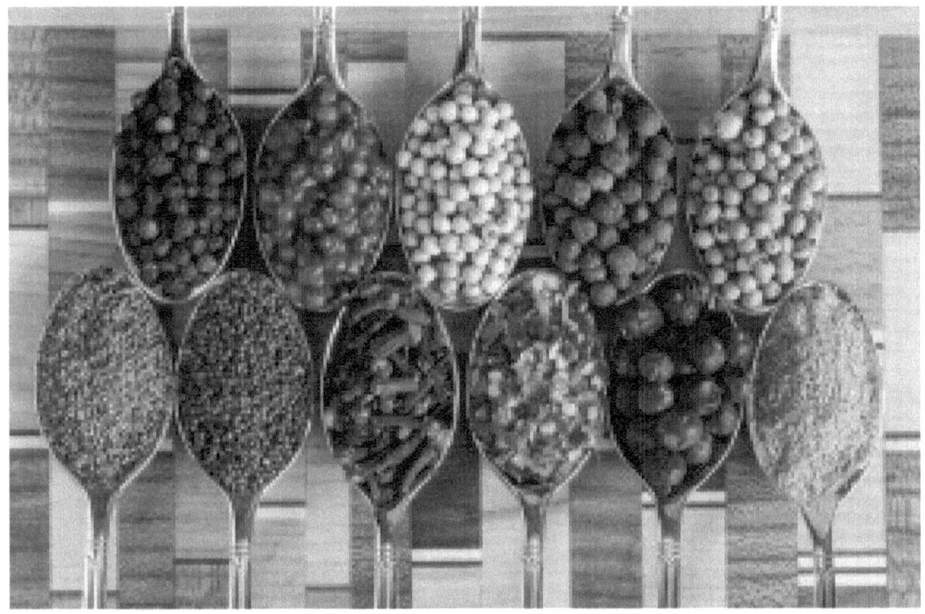

You can include the following condiments to your keto diet plan:

- Pepper
- Herbs
- Salt
- Spices
- Horseradish
- Aioli

MEATS WHICH ARE KETO FRIENDLY

You should avoid all processed meats. It is important that you choose unprocessed meats, as they are mostly keto-friendly and contain fewer carbs. If you want to go for the healthiest option, you need to choose grass-fed and organic meat. However, since a keto diet is not in high protein, but in fat. You do not have to add huge amounts of meat to your diet plan.

When you consume more meat, you end up with excess protein, which is actually more than your body needs. This will push your body out of ketosis as the gluconeogenesis process takes place—converting your proteins into glucose. So, a small to moderate quantity of meat is more than enough for you to stick to your ketogenic diet routine.

It is better to avoid cold cuts, meatballs, and sausages, as all these processed meats often carry added carbs that are not healthy for your body. If you have no other choice and have to buy processed meats, always look for the ingredients. Remember, your carb intake needs to be less than 5 percent.
You need to be careful of the amount that you consume of the following meats:
- White meat
- Turkey
- Chicken
- Pork products
- Ham
- Sausage
- Bacon

- Red meat
- Steak
- Fatty meats

SEAFOOD AND FISH

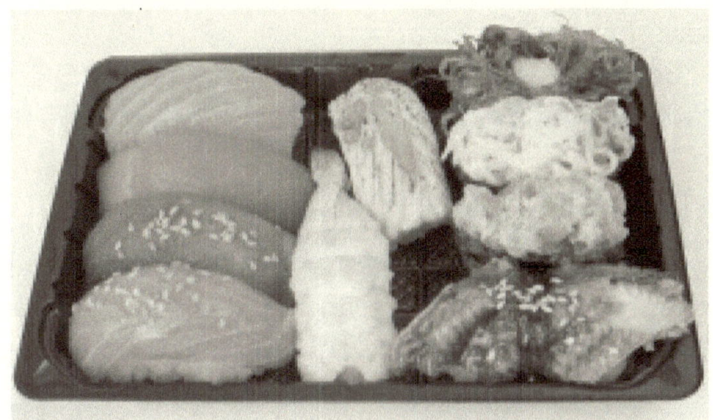

Fatty fish are excellent choices for a good ketogenic diet:
- Tuna
- Salmon
- Mackerel
- Trout

Other seafood, such as shellfish is also a good choice for your keto diet.

EGGS

You can eat them in any form:
- Boiled eggs
- Scrambled eggs
- Omelets
- Fried eggs (with coconut oil or butter)

When you buy eggs, go for omega-3, pastured or free-range eggs (eggs that come from free-range animals). Always choose the organic option! Considering the cholesterol content in eggs, you should not be eating more than 36 eggs in a day, but if you can eat fewer eggs, good for you! When you are making keto-friendly egg recipes, try to add as much unprocessed cheese and butter as possible. It is better to stick to blue cheese, cheddar, or mozzarella.

HIGH-FAT SAUCES, NATURAL FAT

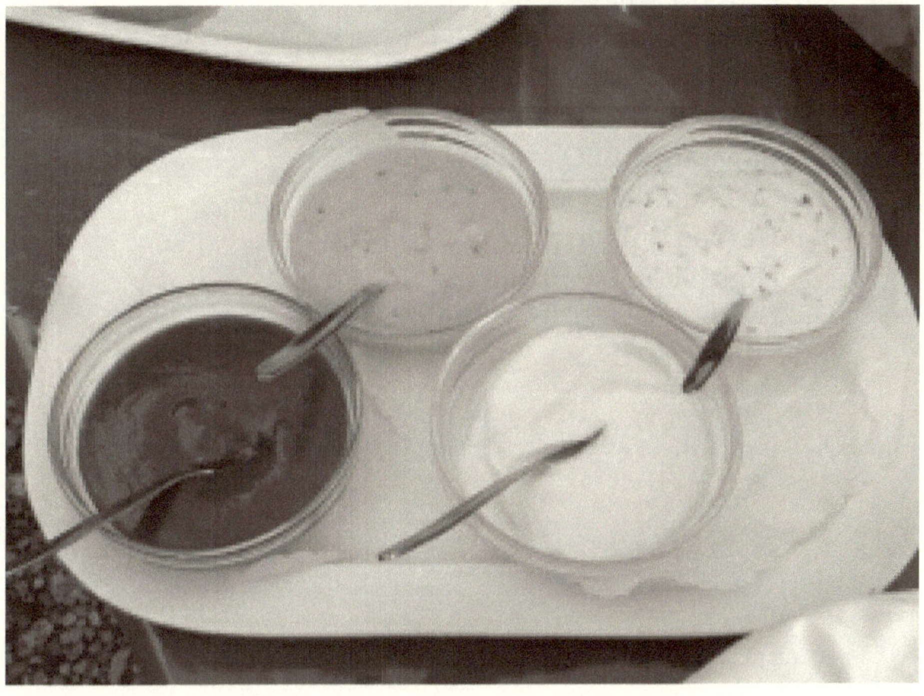

As mentioned earlier, when you are on a keto diet, most of your calories will come from fat, and it is therefore important for you to choose the natural source of fat. Eggs, meat, fish, and seafood are fat-rich food items, but it is also important for you to add more fat to your dishes by cooking in coconut fat, olive oil, coconut oil, butter, etc. You can also include high-fat keto-friendly sauces, dips, and spreads such as:

- Garlic butter
- Béarnaise sauce

- Yellow mustard
- Dijon mustard
- Sriracha mayonnaise
- Full-fat mayonnaise
- Buffalo hot sauce
- Creamy salad dressings
- Pesto
- Alfredo sauce
- Chimichurri
- Nacho cheese sauce
- Tzatziki
- Low-sugar BBQ sauce
- Guacamole
- Herbed butter
- High-fat dairy products

DAIRY

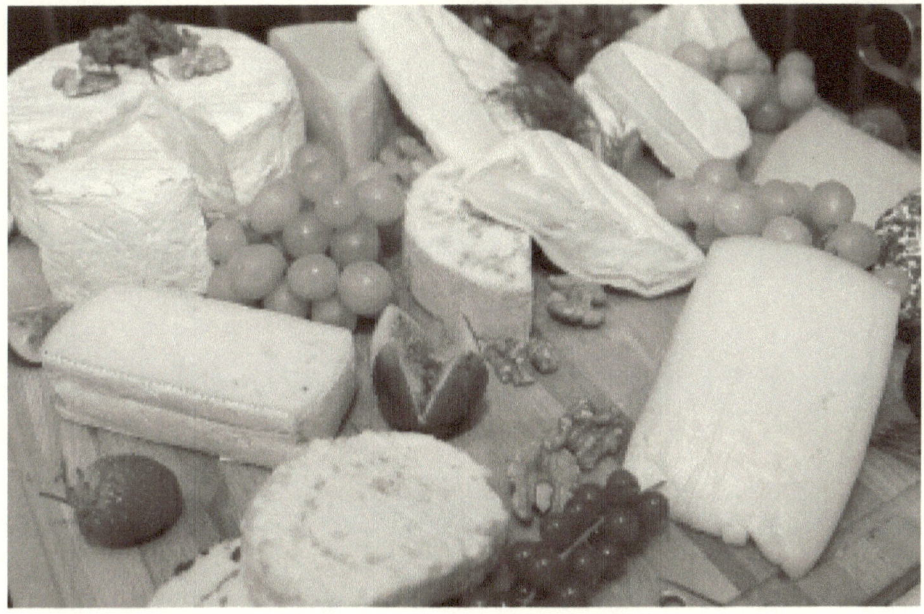

When you are doing your weekly grocery shopping, you probably see many people going for low-fat cheese, low-fat butter, etc.. But in your case, you will have to go for the opposite! The keto diet requires you to add in as much healthy high-fat products as possible, and high-fat dairy is an affordable choice. You can include:

- Heavy cream (for cooking)
- Grass-fed cream and butter
- High-fat unprocessed cheese
- Cheddar
- Mozzarella
- Blue
- Goats cheese (optional)

- High-fat yogurts (don't over-eat)

You can use milk sparingly in your coffee as the milk sugar can add to your carb intake. No cafe, latte, please! When you are not hungry, do not snack on cheese too much as it might interfere with your weight-loss plan.

SIMPLIFIED LIST OF DRINKS THAT ARE ALLOWED ON A KETO DIET

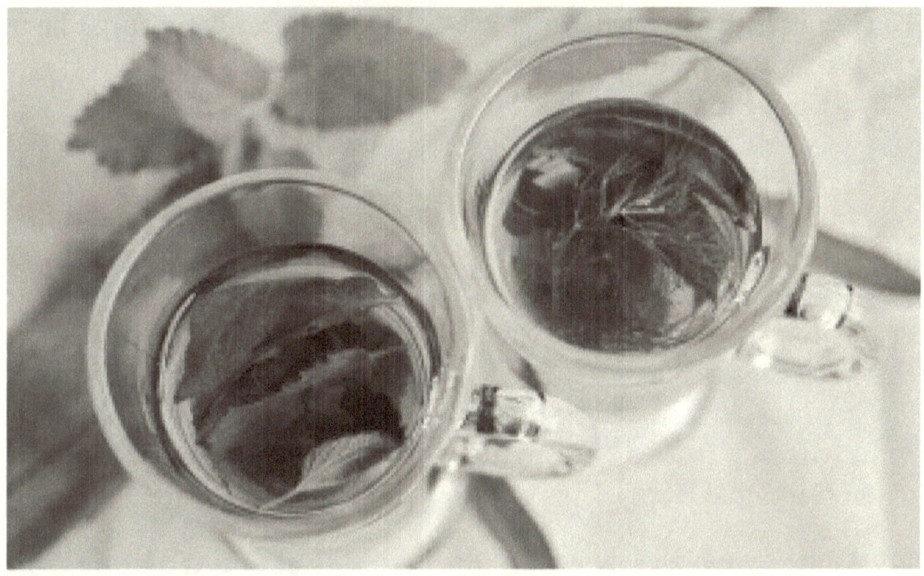

Water is the first option, irrespective of whether you are dieting or not. You need to drink an adequate amount of water to keep your body hydrated. A properly hydrated body will do its work without any hiccups! On a keto diet, you can have:

- Plain water
- Sparkling water
- Iced water
- Hot water
- Naturally flavored water (adding limes, sliced cucum-

> bers, or lemons to your water)
> - Salted water (add half to one tsp. of salt to your drinking water if you are suffering from keto flu symptoms or headaches)

You can drink coffee if you do not add sugar, cream, or milk to it. However, if you are not used to black coffee, you can add a bit of cream or a small amount of milk. You can also turn your coffee into a fat-energized drink by adding coconut oil or butter to it. Also, do not forget to cut back on cream, fat, or milk in your coffee if you feel a lag in your weight-loss timetable.

Tea is another good option, but again, do not add any sugar here too. You can go for the following choices of tea:
- Herbal tea
- Black tea
- Green tea
- Mint tea
- Orange Pekoe tea

Bone broth is yet another drink you can consume on the keto diet. This drink is not only satiating but is also full of electrolytes and nutrients that can keep your body hydrated for hours on end. It is easy to make, and you can add some coconut oil or butter to it for extra energy.

Like your bone broth, vegetable stock is also nutritious. You can make a simple and nutritious stock from mixed vegetables, and you can add more onions and garlic to add a little taste.

Simplified List of Food Items to Avoid on a Keto Diet
When you follow a ketogenic diet, there are some food types that you should avoid. The following list of food items should neither be in your kitchen racks nor on your grocery shopping lists:

SUGAR

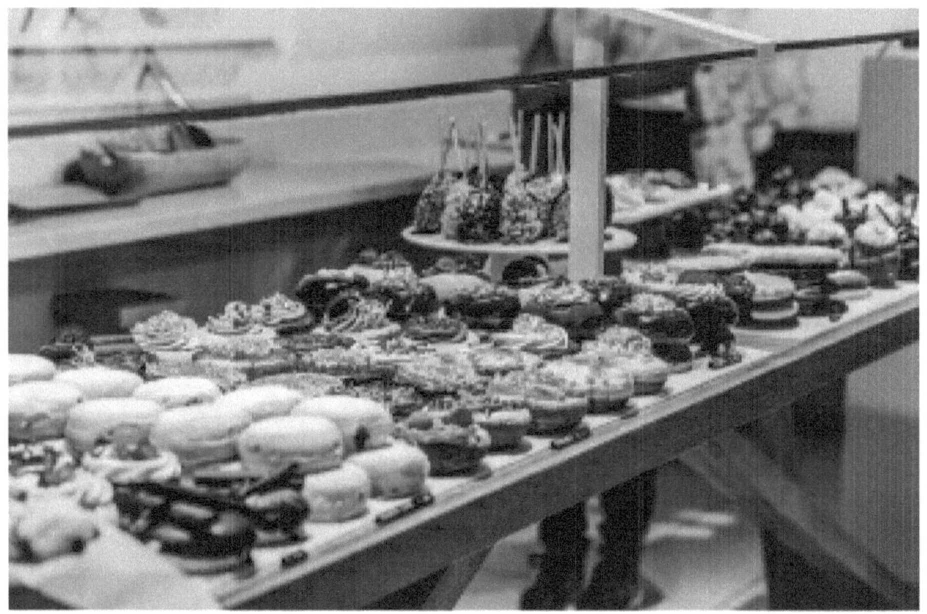

Sugar is the biggest enemy to your keto diet. Get rid of all energy drinks, soft drinks, and vitamin water from your refrigerator —these are all nothing but sugared water. You also need to avoid fruit juices as they have high sugar content. You should also say a big fat NO to the following foods:

- Candy
- Cookies
- Sweets
- Donuts
- Cakes
- Breakfast cereals
- Frozen treats
- Chocolate bars

- Maple syrup
- Agave nectar
- Honey
- Artificial sweeteners (avoid or limit its usage)
- Smoothies
- Ice creams
- Sugary snacks

When you are buying dressing, condiments, packaged food products, drinks, and sauces, ensure to check the label for the carb content and hidden sugars.

STARCH

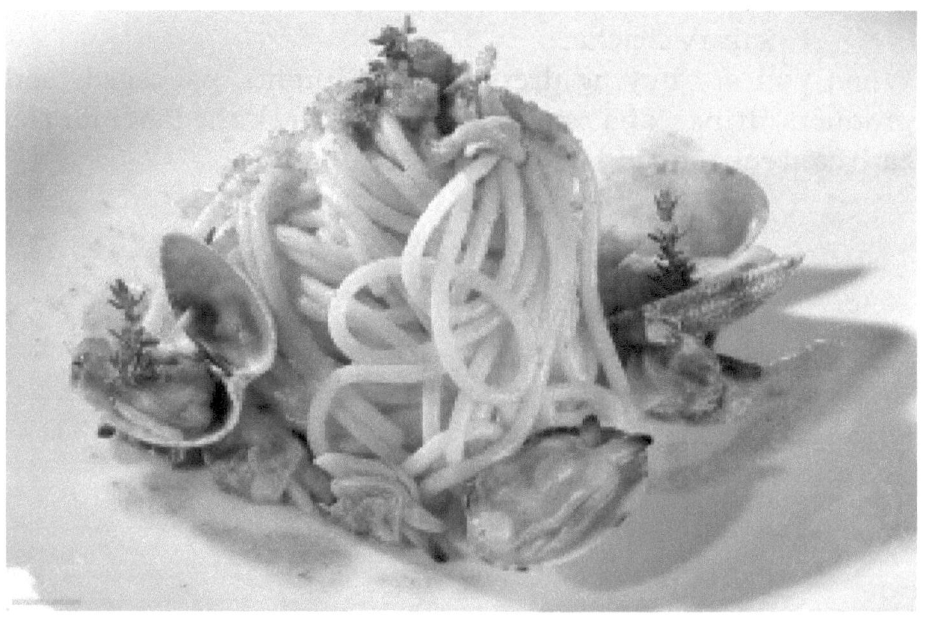

You need to avoid the following carb-rich foods, as they are rich in starch and other not-so-keto-friendly contents:

- Rice
- Bread
- Pasta
- Corn
- Potatoes, in a limited amount (sweet potatoes too)
- Muesli
- Potato chips
- Porridge
- French Fries
- Wholegrain products

You may have seen lentils and beans in the list of foods that you can eat, but you should not overeat them as that may lead to a carb overload.
There is also keto-friendly bread, pasta, rice, and porridge as replacements.

BEER

Beer, also called liquid bread, is rich in carbs. There are too many quickly absorbed carbs in it. Do not worry, as there are a couple of lower-carb beer options! Check this out—https://www.dietdoctor.com/low-carb/keto/alcohol-guide#beer

FRUIT

Avoid fruit, apart from those that have been mentioned in the list of foods that you can eat. Fruit naturally has a high sugar content (fructose), so eating them occasionally is fine.

MARGARINE

Margarine is not butter—it is imitation butter produced by the food industry. It has a high content of omega-6 fat, which is abnormal. It is unhealthy and does not taste good! Margarine is related to various diseases such as allergies, asthma, and inflammatory disorders.

TUBERS AND ROOT VEGETABLES

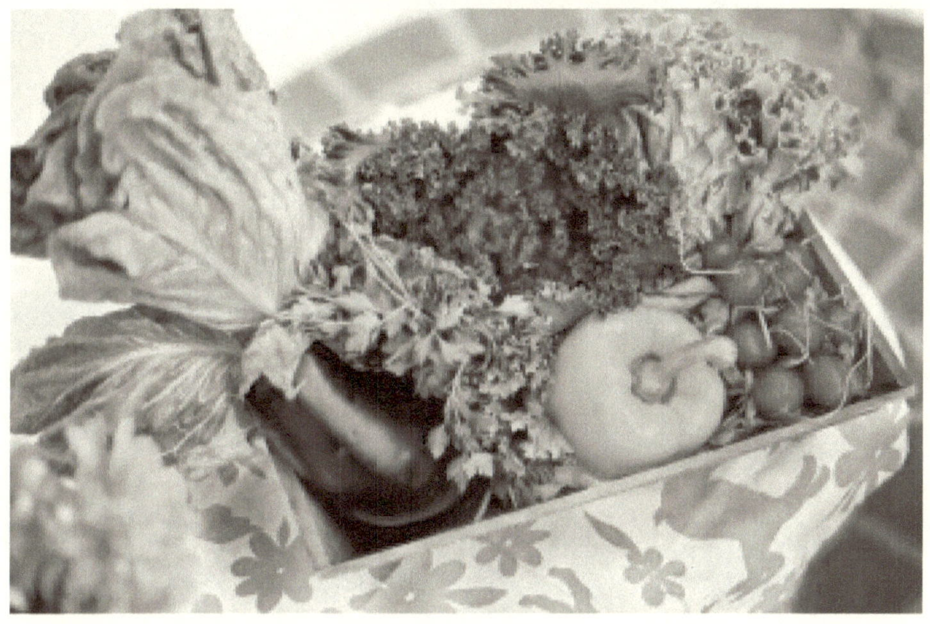

Apart from potatoes and sweet potatoes, you will also need to avoid:

- Parsnips
- Carrots (limited quantity is fine)
- Celery root
- Beets
- *Processed food*
- Low-fat diet products (highly processed and rich in carbs)
- Unhealthy fats (refined oils, processed vegetable oils, mayonnaise, low-fat butter, canola oil, etc.)

- Sauces and Condiments which contain sugar or unhealthy fat
- Sugar-free diet foods (they contain high sugar alcohols that can disturb your state of ketosis. They are also highly processed)
- Alcohol (beverages that has alcohol in them can kick you out of ketosis because they are usually high in carbs)

OTHER KETO-APPROVED FOODS THAT YOU CAN MUNCH ON

You can go ahead and eat the following keto-approved healthy snack items or use them as ingredients for your keto snacks. However, I repeat that you must only indulge in snacking if you are truly hungry between meals.

- A handful of seeds or nuts
- Cheese (couple it up with olives)
- Dark chocolate (90 percent – better to eat the ones that don't have any form of milk content in it)
- One or two hard-boiled eggs
- Strawberries with cream
- Low-carb milkshake (cocoa powder + nut butter + almond milk)
- Full-fat yogurt (blend it with cocoa powder and nut butter)
- Celery with guacamole and salsa
- Small portions of left-over meals

SIMPLIFIED GROCERY SHOPPING LISTS

When starting a new diet, it is quite common to get intimidated. More often than not, people are confused and have no clue where to start! The first step to any diet routine is to:

- Listen to your body and understand what it wants
- Research on what is needed to improve your current health condition
- Focus on your overall wellness

Your grocery-shopping list should only include food that adheres to the keto diet rules. So, remember to remove carb-rich foods from your kitchen cabinet and refrigerator. All processed foods, starchy vegetables, sugar, grains, bread, natural or artificial sweeteners, and sugar-rich drinks should also not be present in your kitchen.

When you start a ketogenic diet, you should include the following protein and produce on your grocery list. You can decide on the quantity based on your week's plan, and do not hesitate to invent your own recipes!

Proteins:
- Tempeh
- Chicken breast/legs
- Beef or pork
- Eggs
- Plain goat milk yogurt

Staples Needed in Your Kitchen:

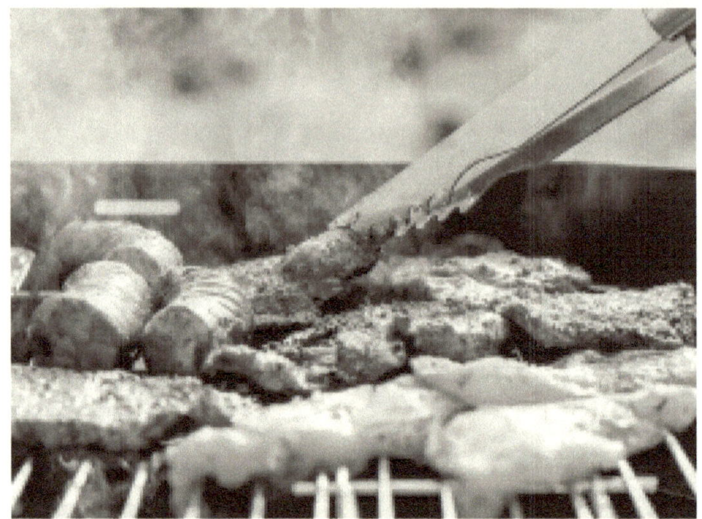

- Coconut cream
- Coconut Aminos
- Cocoa powder
- Vanilla extract
- Almond flour
- Almond butter
- Peanut butter
- Monk fruit extract
- Almond milk (or any preferred nut milk)
- Coconut milk
- Oils and Spices
- Coconut oil
- Olive oil
- Salt (preferably sea salt)
- Pepper
- Ground ginger or ginger powder
- Garlic powder
- Cinnamon powder

Foods Rich in Omega-3 Fatty Acids:
- Sardines
- Flax seeds
- Grass-fed butter
- Cod liver oil

- Algae
- Chia seeds
- Salmon
- Hemp seeds
- Egg yolk
- Grass-fed beef
- Walnuts

Dairy Products:
- Cream cheese
- Cheese (preferably blue cheese, cheddar, or mozzarella)
- Sour cream
- Heavy whipping cream
- Salted butter (preferred)
- Greek Yoghurt (Plain)
- Cottage cheese

Keto-Friendly Sweeteners (one or two of them):
- Monkfruit
- Stevia
- Swerve
- Erythritol
- Allulose
- Truvia
- Sucralose
- Saccharin
- Aspartame

Vegetables

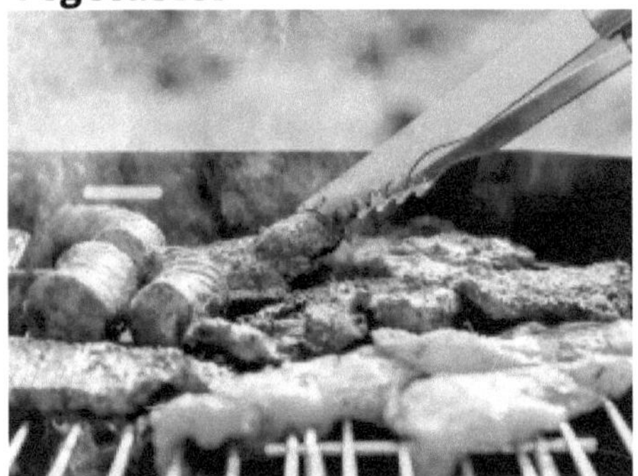

- Mushrooms
- Cabbage
- Cauliflower
- Broccoli
- Brussels sprouts
- Onions
- Spinach
- Celery

- Green beans
- Lettuce
- Asparagus
- Peas
- Kale
- Radishes or turnips
- Garlic
- Artichokes
- Okra
- Tomatoes
- Cucumbers
- Bell peppers
- Eggplant

Fruit

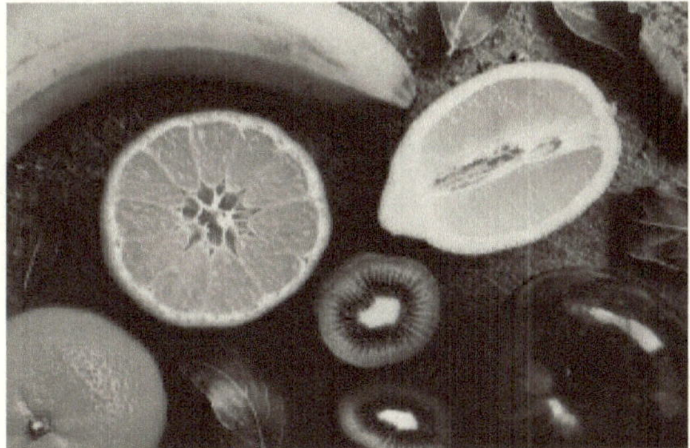

- Berries (choose keto-friendly berries like strawberry, blackberry, raspberry)
- Avocado
- Olives
- Squash
- Lime
- Lemon

TOP MYTHS ABOUT THE KETO DIET

There are many myths about the keto diet that need to be debunked. Unfortunately, because of these myths or misunderstandings, some people feel discouraged to go on this diet. This is why it is important for you to know the truth to make sure that you understand what the keto diet really is. Let's look at the myths one by one:

KETOSIS CAN BE DANGEROUS

Ketosis is the state that you reach when you are on a keto diet, and you should stay in this zone of ketosis for as long as you can, as it is the state where the body is a powerful fat burner. So, is it dangerous? Definitely not. Remember that ketosis is a natural reaction and process of the human body. What is dangerous is not ketosis but ketoacidosis. When you are in ketosis, you are free to leave the state of ketosis at any time you want. You can swiftly do this by consuming more carbs. However, in ketoacidosis, the process becomes uncontrollable. Your blood sugar can spike up, and your body might produce too many ketones. Ketoacidosis is an abnormal response of the body. Still, it is worth noting that as far as ketosis alone is concerned, it is safe.

THE BODY NEEDS LOTS OF CARBOHYDRATES

This is true only if the body does not enter into a state of ketosis. Once the body reaches ketosis, it starts to produce ketones from fats and uses them as an energy source. Studies show that the energy that is supplied to the body when in ketosis is even more effective than that coming from carbohydrates. As you are following a keto diet, you do not need to depend on carbs, as ketones will be your primary source of energy.

FOLLOWING A KETO DIET CAN LEAD TO CLOGGED ARTERIES

This is indeed scary, but it is only a myth. Here is the truth: a true keto diet will not clog your arteries and lead to different heart diseases. On the contrary, the keto diet is good for your body and heart. You need to know that just because a keto diet is a high-fat diet, it does not necessarily mean that you can eat all the bacon that you want. You have to make sure that the bulk of the fats that you consume is good cholesterol. Now, again, do not let the word cholesterol give you a wrong impression. Did you know that the cells in your body need cholesterol to function effectively? Yes, your body needs cholesterol. But then again, you have to be careful with the quality as well as the amount of cholesterol that you feed to your body.

IT IS BAD FOR YOUR KIDNEYS

A diet is only bad for your kidneys if it is high in protein. By now, you should already know that a keto diet is not a high-protein diet, but rather a diet that is moderate in protein. Therefore, it is not bad for your kidneys as long as you stick to the proper proportions and quantities. In fact, research suggests that going on a keto diet for just a few days is beneficial to your kidneys, as well as for other organs.

IT IS BAD FOR YOUR COLON

Just like the myth about it being bad for kidneys, this is not true. Remember that the keto diet is also a diet that is high in fiber, so it is good for your colon. This is because when you are on a keto diet, you are strongly encouraged to consume vegetables such as spinach, cabbage, and many others. Going on this diet is actually good for your colon. In fact, if you are having issues with your colon or any other gastrointestinal matters, then going on a keto diet might be just what you need.

IT WILL CAUSE YOUR MUSCLES TO SHRINK

Remember, the keto diet is a diet that is moderate in protein, so you do not have to be worried about losing muscle. The keto diet recognizes the body's need for protein and makes it a part of this diet. Now, keep in mind that your muscles will only shrink if you do not eat enough protein or if you fail to enter a state of ketosis. Ketosis is the state you will be in once you are on a keto diet, and you will still continue to consume protein. As you can see, you do not have to worry about this myth at all.

FOR THE BRAIN TO FUNCTION EFFECTIVELY, IT NEEDS GLUCOSE FROM CARBS

Again, this is a myth that needs to be debunked. You need to understand that the brain will only need glucose from carbs if and only if it is not in a state of ketosis. Consuming little carbs or even a lack of it will not cause your brain to stop working properly as long as it is powered by ketones. In fact, studies show that the brain functions more effectively when it is powered by ketones. Of course, if you are on a ketogenic diet, then you are in a state of ketosis where you are continuously powered by ketones. Those practicing the keto diet even claim that they experience a sudden increase in mental focus and concentration.

THE KETO DIET WILL ONLY MAKE YOU WEAK

This is probably true at the beginning of the diet when your body is still adjusting to it. However, it is only temporary. In fact, those who have adjusted to the diet claim to have increased their physical performance and endurance. You simply need to give your body enough time to adjust, especially if you are the type who is not used to being on a low-carb diet. Just be kind and patient to yourself as you allow your body to get used to this healthy diet. Soon enough, you will start to feel more energized, and you will not worry about feeling weak.
Page Break

HOW TO GET STARTED WITH KETO

Getting Started on a Keto Diet

Now that you have a full understanding of what the keto diet is and the foods you can and can't eat, you can get started. Many people find it hard to get started with a new diet, especially when there are too many rules and instructions involved. Each diet tells you something different to do, and it can be confusing.

The ketogenic diet, on the other hand, is very easy to follow. The basic rule of thumb is to avoid factory-processed food and to eat wholesome meals.

Any packaged and commercially sold food items will have many hidden ingredients that you aren't really aware of. These will include sugars, preservatives, additives, etc. that are all unhealthy for you. A glass of soda will usually have more sugar than your required dietary allowance, and more often than not you tend to drink a few glasses a day. Sugar itself is a very bad ingredient in your diet and should cut it off as soon as possible. Processed foods with sugar are one of the main causes of weight gain and obesity. Even if what you buy is not sweet, sugar might still be an ingredient, just in another form.

When you buy a processed product, check the labels for ingredients every time.

You might not realize it, but pizza also contains sugar. On labels, sugar is written in different names. There are many products on the market with sugar in them, so it is not surprising that obesity has been increasing at an alarming rate every year. The keto diet just helps you understand what is healthy and unhealthy for your body so that you can make better choices. While other diets will tell you to lose weight by not eating much, the keto diet will help you eat and still lose weight.

The easiest way to avoid hidden ingredients like colorants, preservatives, and sugars is to buy raw ingredients or even grow them. The list of foods to avoid and eat will be helpful during your grocery trips. Farmers' markets are a good way to buy organic produce that is healthy for you. Avoid ingredients that are high in carbs like potatoes, even if it's your favorite vegetable. If you always eat bread or some grain with your regular meals, you need to remember that they will only make you gain weight. It is crucial to stop eating more than 20 grams of carbs every day while you follow a ketogenic diet. If you have foods with too many carbs, your body will find it harder to go into the state of ketosis, and the diet will not work for you. Replace these parts of your meal with healthier substitutes. If you really need bread, use almond flour to bake healthier bread. There are healthier alternatives to many foods that are not keto-friendly. The oils that you use for cooking or as dressing for a salad should also be keto-friendly. Don't worry; they will still taste just as good. Cooking with butter can actually make most dishes taste richer and more flavorful. Who knew butter was good for you? Olive oil and walnut oil are much healthier than most seed oils that you usually use.

To get started, there are a few examples of meals that you can prepare on a keto diet. This will provide you with a starting point, but there are many more recipes that you can try each and every day while you stay on the ketogenic routine. The first step is to be determined that you want to achieve a certain goal. Get rid of any food in the house that is not keto-friendly. Buy all the healthy ingredients recommended above and stock your pantry. Start trying out new recipes to make it a fun transition.

The first week or so can be a little difficult, and you might notice some side effects. Before you begin, get a check-up, and ask your doctor if the diet is suitable for you. If you get their approval, the common side effects are just temporary and will pass. You can even take precautions and avoid symptoms like dizziness, dehydration, etc. If something seems too unnatural to you, just consult your doctor again. A few supplements and a lot of water usually do the trick. You need to persevere through the initial adaptation stage and let your body get used to the new diet. Soon, your system will get used to the keto-genic foods and act accordingly. As your body starts going into ketosis, you will start burning stored fat and lose weight. Usually, your body will help you lose weight until it reaches an appropriate number and then maintain it.

The moment you feel that you are losing too much weight, you can always adjust your diet accordingly. For those who exercise regularly, it is not necessary to load up on carbs, as fats will also provide you with the energy you need. If your activities are too intense, you can add a little more carbohydrate if your trainer recommends it. The keto diet is good enough, regardless of what else you do.

You need to remember that everyone's body is different and will react differently. The diet might work better for some people and help them lose weight faster, while the process might be slower for others. This will just be determined by the individual, and neither is right or wrong. The keto diet will work slowly and help you achieve a healthy weight and help you maintain it. It is not a fad diet that will make you skinny through starvation. If you don't notice any changes over a long time, you might not be following the diet properly. It is important to reduce carbs, keep proteins moderate, eat a lot of fat and cut out all manufactured products. The diet will help you if you help yourself. A cheat day is allowed once in a while, but if you do it too often, the diet won't work. If you really want to lose weight, I recommend avoiding cheat days until you've at least reached your weight goal. Eating junk food once in a while can also shake your resolve to stick to the diet, and all your effort will be in vain. Stick to the list of keto foods and watch it work for you. Adding some regular exercise will help it work better for you, but it is not a compulsory requirement of the keto diet.

KETO, STEP-BY-STEP

So, if you already decided to go on a ketogenic diet, good for you. The keto diet is an awesome diet that will make you healthy, fit, and strong. If this is your first time going on a healthy diet, then expect it to be quite an adventure. Now, regarding the keto diet, you should understand that it can be quite challenging to reach the state of ketosis for the first time. It takes a few days before you can reach this state, but it is well worth every effort you put into it. As the body adjusts to the diet, it will be easier. You just have to be patient and get used to it.

Okay, so now you know that a keto diet is low in carbs, moderate in protein, and high in fats. But what does this mean, exactly? So that you can properly get on the keto diet, it is important that you formulate a plan. It is best that you keep your plan simple. After all, going on keto does not need to be a complicated process. If you think that dropping your carb intake drastically is hard for you, do it gradually. This is a good way to adjust from your old unhealthy diet into a new healthy keto diet. If you are used to a high-carb diet, suddenly restricting your carb intake can be really difficult. So, feel free to take it easy on yourself, but be sure to work on sticking to the keto diet and aim for continuous improvement.

However, if you think that you already have what it takes to be on a full keto diet, then you can drop your carb intake significantly right away. Although this is easy, it is the fastest way to get into the state of ketosis, which is the state that you need to be in on a ketogenic diet.

Knowing what keto diet is composed of is still not enough. Let us get into more specific details so that you know just how to plan your diet. Let us discuss the foods that you should eat:

Meat

Meat is not only tasty, but it is also an excellent source of protein. You should stick to meat that is low in carbs like fish, beef, and eggs. Do not forget that the keto diet is a diet that is moderate in the consumption of meat, so be careful not to eat more than you should.

Vegetables

Vegetables are part of the keto diet. In essence, it is strongly encouraged to eat vegetables. After all, they are very nutritious, which makes them good for your health. Stick to green and leafy vegetables like spinach and kale. You can also eat cauliflower, broccoli, and other ground vegetables.

High-Fat Dairy

Foods that are high in fat are a staple part of your keto diet. Of course, you cannot just eat any fatty foods. You should choose healthy dairy foods that are high in fat, such as butter, cream, and cheese, among others.

Seeds and Nuts

Seeds and nuts like almonds, sunflower seeds, macadamia, and others are rich in nutrients. They are also an excellent snack when you are feeling hungry.

Strawberries and Other Berries

Eating berries is a good way to satisfy your sweet tooth. Eat healthy berries like blackberries, strawberries, kiwis, and others.

Sweetener

If you want to use a sweetener, use one that has a low carbohydrate content like Splenda.

Other Fats

Excellent and healthy sources of fats include salad dressing, coconut oil, and saturated fats. It is important to know this since the keto diet is high in fats. In a keto diet, you can eat bacon, but you are encouraged to choose healthier fat options. When you're feeling hungry, you might want to eat peanut butter, cheese, and nuts, among others, instead.

Water

If you choose to go on a keto diet, water is your best friend. Water is a natural cleansing agent, and it can also help you deal with your hunger pangs. You can also add salt to water to increase your electrolytes. Also, you should learn to distinguish being hungry from being thirsty. Many people eat when, in fact, they just need to drink water. This can help you keep your carb count low.

Page Break

THE RESULTS OF THE KETO DIET

According to studies, people following the ketogenic diet experience a decrease in their overall body weight. Experts conducted further research and clinical trials to better understand the ketogenic diet. They found that:

- When you eat carbs, your body tends to retain the fluid to store the carbs as a reserve for energy (just in case your body needs it in the future).

- Now, when you minimize or eliminate the carb intake, this fluid does not have much use, so you lose this water weight.

- People often overeat when they consume a large quantity of carbohydrates. When you follow a high-carb diet, you eat more since you are always craving food. However, when you consume a high-fat diet, you feel full, and your cravings reduce. The moment you are on a ketogenic diet, your body depletes its entire carb reserves and looks for an alternate energy source. Your body shifts into ketosis and targets the stored fat to produce energy, thereby reducing your body weight.

People started to accept this new low-carb high-fat diet because the diet protocol made sense to many. Most people will want to lose some fat from their body to achieve their goal weight, and this diet does exactly that by converting the stored fat to a fuel source.

KETOSIS AND HOW IT WORKS

The Ketogenic diet, commonly known as the keto diet, is a dietary protocol that expects you to focus on increasing your fat intake and eliminating or reducing your carb intake. This will push your body to a certain metabolic state known as ketosis. The moment your body enters into a state of ketosis, it converts the stored fat to fuel and burns it to provide energy to your cells. So, when you are in ketosis, your body burns the stored and dietary fat for fuel, and eventually, you reach your goal of losing weight, getting healthy, looking good, and feeling lighter!

For this to happen, your body should exhaust all the glycogen (stored glucose–sugar) reserves from your body. How do you make this happen?

- You can put your body into the state of ketosis when you undergo a complete fast, i.e. you do not eat anything at all, thereby giving no calories to your body. As this takes place, your body does not get any new glucose and therefore turns to its reserve—glycogen (stored glucose). It depletes the entire glucose stores and then starts looking for an alternate energy source. This is when it focuses its attention on the stored fat thereby burning it to produce ketone bodies for fuel.

- Another way to put your body into ketosis is by mimicking fasting. You should deprive your body of glucose by eliminating any food that the body can convert into sugar. This is possible when you increase your fat intake and reduce or eliminate your carb intake. In other words, you deny your body of glucose, thereby forcing it to look for an alternate energy resource–fat.

When you look at a typical American diet, you will find that it has more than 50 percent carbohydrates, and this is why over 60 percent of the country is obese or overweight. When you replace the carbs with another fuel source, you start to burn fat. Eliminating the carbs or reducing the intake of carbs drastically can make this happen! A ketogenic diet implies a dietary approach, which is moderate in protein, high in fat intake, and has a minimal to no intake of carbohydrates.

When you practice fasting for an extended period or when you consume foods that adhere to the ketogenic diet protocol, your body gets into ketosis, thereby forcing it to burn all the stored fats for fuel.

Another important thing is that when you eat carb-rich foods, your body produces insulin to manage the glucose (sugar) increase in your bloodstream. So naturally, when you reduce the consumption of carbs, the insulin production reduces, thus making your body more insulin sensitive. This comes with a multitude of health benefits.

So, when your body shifts into ketosis, you not only lose weight but also experience:
- Lower insulin levels
- Increased energy
- More physical potential
- Increased cognitive ability and brain function

KETONES

So, what exactly are these ketones, and where do they come from? As mentioned earlier, when your body exhausts its glucose reserves (glycogen), it will look for another alternative energy source. This is when it starts digging into the body's fat storehouse as stored fat can help to fuel the required energy for your cells.

Since there is no glucose in the body, your liver will take in the stored fats and convert them into fatty acids. These fatty acids are then simplified into functional compounds known as ketone bodies (otherwise known as ketones). Your body uses these ketones to provide energy to your body and brain cells. The best part is that when your blood ketone levels increase, your appetite decreases. The reason for improved energy is that your brain uses a different source to produce energy.

Your liver generates three different types of ketone bodies:
- Acetoacetate
- Beta-Hydroxybutyrate
- Acetone

Your body can fuel itself from ketones in two different ways:

- The body is in a position to make its own ketones when you fast or when you increase your fat intake and reduce your carb intake, forcing the abstinence of glucose
- You can also feed your body with actual ketones by consuming exogenous ketones (ketone supplements)

When your body is on a ketogenic diet, it acts as a fat-burning machine as it shifts its chief energy source from glucose to stored fat. This naturally leads to low insulin levels, and the fat-burning power increases as accessing the stored fat becomes easy. Your body is in ketosis when it produces ketones, and the fastest way to shift your body into ketosis is by fasting. But it is impossible to fast forever, and this led to the development of the ketogenic diet.

Is it possible to lose weight when the body enters into ketosis?
When your body begins to burn stored fat into ketones, your body shifts into ketosis. But you might be wondering: "Why will that make me reduce weight?" I understand where you are coming from. Let me explain this to you with an example.

Imagine you have stored a pile of coal for the upcoming winter. When it is winter, you scoop up some of these coal piles into the furnace for heat. As you continue to use up the coal, the pile gets smaller. Similarly, in ketosis, your body burns the stored fat in your body, and as it continues to utilize the stored fats (which is your extra flab, water weight, excess calories, etc.), you get smaller, i.e. you reduce weight. The coal here is the stored fat, and the heat you receive in winter is your energy.

There are numerous studies showing how a well-planned ketogenic diet has helped countless people to lose weight and improved their overall health condition by improving their health markers. Another important reason for losing weight on the ketogenic diet is thermodynamics! When you practice the keto diet, you are getting rid of one major macronutrient—carbohydrates.

The following list includes food items that are rich in carbohydrates.
- Soda
- Bagels
- Fruit smoothies
- Bread
- Sugar candies

- White rice
- Pasta

These foodstuffs are high in caloric value, and when you over-eat, these carbs are stored in your body as fat. When you restrict or eliminate these carb-rich foods, you consume fewer calories. When you burn more calories than you consume, you lose weight. This is why most calorie-restricted diets result in weight loss when done right, regardless of the proportion of food you consume. On this type of diet, you are not concentrating on body composition, food quality, or muscle synthesis, but rather on the amount of food consumption (smaller portions of food).

When your body gets adapted to the keto routine, you feel satiated with fewer calories, which ultimately results in losing weight easier and quicker. But remember, if you overeat on a keto diet, you will definitely gain more weight. So, do not expect to lose weight after eating 6000 calories of bacon, beef, and butter regularly! You should know how to eat healthily!

The ketogenic diet not only helps with weight loss but also aids in:

- Treatment of epilepsy
- Type 2 diabetes
- Managing PCOS (Polycystic ovary syndrome)
- Treatment of acne
- Showing improvement in neurological diseases such as MS (multiple sclerosis and Parkinson's)
- Reducing the risk of cardiovascular and respiratory diseases

Scientists are conducting more research to understand how the keto diet affects patients with Alzheimer's and similar health conditions.

HOW TO CHECK THE RESULTS OF A KETO DIET

If you want to check whether your body has entered a state of ketosis, there are certain tools that can help you measure it.

I. The first is urine strips that are easily available, and they're an affordable option. You just have to dip the urine strip in your urine. The color change is used to indicate the presence of ketones in your urine. If the reading on the strip is high or the darkest color, then you know that your body is undergoing ketosis.

II. Ketone breath analyzers are another option. These are much more expensive than urine strips but are reusable, unlike the latter. There is no precise marker for the level of ketones in your breath, but using a color code, the analyzer helps to check if they are present or not.

III. The most expensive tool to measure ketosis is the blood ketone meter. This is the most precise equipment to measure the presence and level of ketones in your blood. The only disadvantage of blood ketone meters is that they are extremely expensive; however, these days, there are cheaper tests available.

Any of the above tools can be used if you want to check the presence of ketones in your body and learn if the process of ketosis has begun. This can be an encouraging way to stick to the diet and continue the diet to lose weight.

Another thing that you can take note of is how to know if your body is at the optimal level of ketosis. Blood ketone meters have very specific markings that will help you out with this aspect. If the level is below 0.5 mmol/l, then this is not ketosis, but you are getting close to it; however, this low level will never help you burn fat in your body. In the initial stage, you might find the level to be between 0.5 mmol/l and 1.5 mmol/l. This is a lower level of ketosis which is beneficial but still not optimal for the kind of results you want. Optimal ketosis occurs between 1.5 and 3 mmol/l. This level is recommended to see the maximum results from ketosis.

At this level, ketosis will result in burning a lot of the excess fat stored in your body, and it will speed up the process of weight loss.

When you enter this state, you will notice that your mental and physical performance is getting better. If your blood ketone level is more than 3 mmol/l, it is higher than recommended. You will not get any special results compared to the optimal level, so don't try to push your body to this state. This level usually indicates that you have not been eating enough, and it is called starvation ketosis. Those who suffer from type 1 diabetes often experience this due to a lack of insulin. The most dangerous level is 8-10 mmol/l, which is a very uncommon, bad ketone count. Most of the time, it is associated with Type I diabetes and has severe symptoms like nausea, abdominal pain, confusion, etc. You will feel very unwell if your ketone levels are this high, and it can even be fatal, so you should seek immediate medical attention.

The blood ketone meter can be a very useful tool to check if you are going about your diet in the right way. Don't over-do it and try to slowly push your body into ketosis. Also, don't try to starve yourself to achieve weight loss faster. This does not work with the ketogenic diet and is against its principles. Allow the diet to work for you by following all its guidelines.

Achieving the optimal blood ketone level is your aim, and you should work to maintain it when you get there. Don't assume that higher ketone levels will help you burn even more fat and lose weight. You should not lose weight at the detriment of your health. Your goal is to lose weight in a healthy way to improve the mental and physical state of your body. If you follow the ketogenic diet in the right way, you will definitely achieve this.

HOW THE KETO DIET LEADS TO WEIGHT LOSS

The foods in the ketogenic diet are important because they begin the process of ketosis and your ability to use fat for energy creation. It is important to understand that you have chosen a diet that requires you to count calories. For some people, this can be tough as it is time-consuming. However, if you can learn to love counting calories, it will be much easier for you.

An overweight person of five foot two should eat 1200 to 1400 calories if they are sedentary or attempt moderate exercise. It also depends on the person's health issues. For example, females battle with hypothyroidism, which is a lack of thyroid secretory hormone (TSH), which is necessary for metabolism, skin, hair, and other endocrine functions. When a person does not have enough TSH, T3, and T4 production, they can gain weight, lose hair, have extremely dry skin, become extremely cold, lethargic, and depressed. With proper hormone regulation, a person suffering from this disease can lose weight, feel happy, and feel better overall.

The ketogenic diet is great for people like this because it requires moderation in food, and in particular, many people with hypothyroidism find that carbs prevent proper metabolism from occurring.

Based on this example, you can see why it is important to speak with a physician before starting any new diet. You want to address any health concerns and discover the optimal daily caloric intake for you and your body type.
Someone who is over six feet tall will naturally require more

calories to sustain a normal healthy body while dieting.

COUNTING CALORIES

Once you know the proper amount of food to eat for your body height and weight, when trying to lose weight, you can begin setting up meals.

You have a couple of options, such as going for three large meals, three small meals, and two snacks, or "grazing" throughout the day with your calorie target in mind.

The key is not when you eat, as long as you ensure you do not feel starving. There is one caveat to "when" you eat. For over ten years, doctors have agreed that eating after 8 p.m. is not conducive to weight loss unless you work nights. For a person who has a 9-5 job, and goes to bed around 9 p.m. to 11 p.m., eating after 8 p.m. does not provide your body enough time to metabolize the food, particularly because you are often sedentary by that time of night.

Today, there are tools to make it easier for you to count calories. Many online websites have popped up where people have put the nutritional information for food from the grocery store and top chain restaurants. All you need to do is create a profile to look at all the food menus you like. The best part is that these websites have apps for your phone, so you can enter what you are eating throughout the day to maintain your caloric intake.

You can also monitor your weight loss by adding your weight every day. When you weigh yourself, it is best done in the morning, every day, at the same time before you eat or drink, as your weight can vary depending on how much you drink and if you are retaining water.

You also want to mentally keep track of bowel movements to

ensure you are having at least one regular movement per day. This is your waste management, and if you are constipated or not getting rid of waste, you are naturally going to weigh more. This has to do with the ease of emptying your bladder when it is blocked.

A secondary tool to purchase is a ketogenic recipe book with a calorie counter and food suggestions. You may need a couple of books. For example, there is an option to find a calorie counter that lists every fruit, vegetable, meat, dairy, and food known to humans. It provides you with the "bad" and "good" carbs, as well as fat, protein, and other nutrition information to help you choose from the "good" list of foods.

Finally, if you have a slow metabolism, it's advised to eat 46 grams of carbs or less per day. The ketogenic diet will have you cutting out carbs altogether or eating fewer than 23 grams per day, which is great.

CHAPTER 5: KETO MEAL PREP AND PLAN

It is unfortunate to say, but sometimes we are so busy to think of what we want or should eat, let alone what we should cook. It is not very easy to eat healthy foods if you lead a busy life unless you have everything planned. *Deciding what to eat every day can, sadly, be a source of stress.* What you will cook for dinner or what you will eat for breakfast or lunch can get tiring, especially if you are on a healthy lifestyle.

Now, imagine for someone who is on a diet such as the keto diet, which demands that you have to eat particular foods for the right nutrition to power your body with sufficient energy! While many of us aspire to live healthy lifestyles and set goals to eat healthy, it is never easy following through, and consistency is a big problem. In fact, it is something as simple as having the right meals to eat, which makes many of us fall off the wagon. This is why meal prepping is a great concept for those on the ketogenic diet.

The idea is based on the fact that most weight gain and fat accumulation in the body is as a result of high carbs intake. Carbohydrates are converted into glycogen and fat by the body. The glycogen is stored in the muscles, and the leftover converted carbs are stored as fat.

When the body is starved of new carbs, it burns up the glycogen stored in the muscles. Once exhausted, the body resorts to the fat reservoir for energy. It is for this reason that the ketogenic diet is so popular and is the most recommended diet for weight loss. It is essentially weight loss without opting out of some foods. You can eat virtually anything you want as long as it fits into the diet.

Ketosis has proven to have a variety of health benefits, which include weight loss, blood sugar regulation, disease management (diabetes, high blood pressure, cholesterol issues, etc.), and enhanced mental performance. Ketosis starves your body of carbohydrates, which the liver converts to glucose—reduced glucose means the body burns fat for energy.

Back to the topic at hand. *Meal prepping simply means preparing whole meals ahead of schedule so that they are available for you to eat when the time comes.* This concept is ideal for the busy lifestyle and has gained popularity with people for the amazing time-saving benefits and other benefits, which we will discuss later.

Apart from having ready meals, this concept ensures that you eat reduces portion to help you reach your dieting goals. No more fast food because prepping guarantees that you eat more nutritious meals and no more late-night meals because you always have a ready dish.

The good thing about meal prepping is that you customize it to fit your availability and needs. There is no standard method of doing it. Choose the day to prep your meals and switch it if you have to.

What about if you are reading this and you are not on a keto diet? Well, meal prepping is still something you should consider for the many benefits on offer. Everyone wants an easier life; therefore, meal planning can be adopted by all of us. Meal prep is not only for those on a keto diet; it can be adapted to fit any diet and lifestyle to guarantee that you will have a meal ready for you ahead of time.

By the end of this chapter, you will be well informed about meal prepping in general but, more specifically, keto meal prep.

Meal prepping will simplify your life, save you a lot of time and money, and ensure that you live the healthy lifestyle you want by keeping you on track as far as eating healthy meals is concerned.

The answer to eating what you want affordably and without putting so much time and energy into cooking is meal prepping, and we shall give you great insights and share with you some great recipes to start you off.

Enjoy this introduction to meal prepping, the great recipes, and many other tips.

We have touched on the meaning of a meal prep plan in the introduction and stated that it means to prepare meals in advance. *For the ketogenic diet, meal planning can be defined more specifically to mean preparing full meals in advance using keto-approved ingredients, calories, and recipes so that you have meals ready to eat that meet the requirements of keto,* usually for a week.

The common and most convenient keto meal prep plan runs for a week. In other words, you will prepare meals for a whole week in advance on a designated day. Think about it, in one week, you will need twenty-one meals if you take three meals a day as you should. Thinking of the over-twenty meals daily or at mealtime is hard and is even more exhausting when you have to factor in the nutrition values of every meal because of the keto diet.

Keto meal planning is the way to solve the problem of cooking time, which can be hard to come by during the week, and will ensure that you eat the correct nutrients. More importantly, it is a flexible process that is owned by everyone in his or her own way so that one's needs, preferences, and schedule are conveniently accommodated.

WHY YOU NEED A KETO MEAL PREP PLAN

You know well that a keto diet requires certain amounts of nutrients, mainly carbohydrates, fat, and proteins per meal. Without proper planning, you can never eat right if you are on keto. Therefore, meal prepping ensures that you reach and maintain your dietary goals throughout the week by preventing you from making bad choices during the week.

Remember, for every meal you eat on a keto diet, you need a calorie breakdown as of 5% carbs, 75% fat, and 20% protein. How can you possibly achieve or ensure this every time without effective planning? Keto meal prep planning makes it possible to allocate one day to cook all the foods you will eat throughout the week and use the time you would otherwise spend cooking or thinking of what to cook on other things. A time-saver!

Meal prep will allow you to tailor-make meals to meet your keto needs. It is important to keep in mind that it is a process that will take time to learn but will simplify your routine if you stick to it.

REASONS FOR KETO MEAL PREP PLANNING

Motivation alone is not enough for dieting or losing weight because you will never be motivated every time. There are times when your motivation will be shaken. However, researchers have found that planning is a better factor for dieting and weight-loss success.

Moreover, there are other benefits to meal planning, which include the following:

- Less stress and time deciding what to eat

- Saves time and money

- Helps you achieve dieting needs

How Long Does It Take to Meal-Prep?

To be honest and objective, the duration you take for meal prepping will depend on you and for a variety of reasons, the main one being your preferences and speed. There are other things you need to do, like shopping for the ingredients you will need for your meals. However, *generally, it takes about an hour to cook meal preps for a week.*

The best time to plan and prep your keto meals would be a Saturday or Sunday when most of us have a bit of a break from the rigors of work. Shopping in the afternoon is a good idea because you will not have to deal with the morning rush, keeping in mind that part of the reason why we are prepping is to reduce stress. You should be as relaxed and organized as possible with shopping.

Therefore, the best time to plan or decide the meals for the week would be Saturday morning before you go shopping. That means that you will have a designated time on Sunday to prep your dishes. The key to getting meal planning and prepping right is to pick a time that will be devoid of distraction or interruptions so that you can use the hour you have for cooking efficiently and optimally.

A distraction-free meal planning session is especially important for those who are starting out on keto meal prep planning. Once you are accustomed to the process, planning and prepping times will be reduced considerably. Find the best times that work for you.

A ketogenic diet requires prepping and planning because if you do not get the meals right, you will destabilize the body chemistry. To ease the process of keto meal prep, start with a week's meal plan, pick out the dishes you want for every one of the three meals per day. From the meals you have chosen, you will draw a detailed shopping list ahead of the shopping time so that you will spend as little time as possible buying them and have enough time for preparation.

The ketogenic diet meal prep plan is ideal for the busy person on the ketogenic diet who hardly ever has enough time to prepare his or her meals. If you leave for work early and are back home to sleep most of the week and you are on the keto diet, there is no better option to ensure that you keep on track despite your hectic schedule.

THE BENEFITS OF A KETO DIET MEAL PREP PLAN

- *It eliminates the temptation to eat off-diet.*

Remember that you are on a diet. The keto diet is calories – and nutrients-specific, such that if you falter, you are likely to destabilize your body chemistry and reverse the gains you have made.

Keto meal prepping eliminates the temptation to eat fast food or any other meals that are not healthy since you have your meals prepared beforehand. With meal planning and prepping, the foods you eat will meet your dietary needs because they are well thought out, planned, and prepped in advance. All you will need to do is warm the food and eat it.

- *Keto meal planning and prepping saves time.*

Meal planning and prepping will save you time all round. You save time with shopping since you have a list of everything you want early enough. You save time with cooking since the ingredients are prepared early, and you save time on deciding what to eat.

Consequently, you have more time to assign to other things, like spending time with family and friends, pursuing a hobby, or beating a deadline at work. You save a lot of time you would have spent cooking, shopping, and deciding meals.

- ***Grocery shopping is made easy.***

Meal planning ensures that you know beforehand what you will require for your meals so that you do not leave out anything from your grocery shopping list or struggle to list items down at the last minute. The best way of detailing your shopping list is by sectionalizing the items into the various food categories, such as dairy, grains, fats, fruits, frozen foods, proteins, and veggies.

Always try to get a new food item each week for each category. If you bought tilapia last week for protein, get salmon this week. If you bought broccoli, get cauliflower this week. The list of items you buy must take into account the ketogenic diet nutritional requirement.

- ***It makes meal decision-making easier and reduces stress.***

As many of you may know, settling on what to eat every day three times a week can be difficult and stressful. With keto meal prepping and planning, this problem will be completely eliminated because you do not have to make the decision every day—the decision about what to eat is made once for the whole week. The time you spend preparing your meals is significantly reduced because everything is planned ahead.

The stress that comes with deciding meals and keeping up with the requirements of your keto diet regime will also fizzle away with meal prepping. You will have a calmer and healthier mental predisposition and keep stress-related health problems at bay.

- ***Keto meal prep planning saves money.***

Buying food items for your cooking in bulk saves you a lot of money. No impulse buying, no cases of buying the wrong ingredients because you will know exactly what to buy in advance. Pricing food items ahead brings in the effective element of cost control through portion control. You save money because you will not be eating out every time and will be buying items at a bargain.

Additionally, you will know the right quantities to buy, which will save you from the financial losses incurred through wastes, especially when you buy more than you need and have to throw away what is left or watch it go bad. You also save money by making fewer trips to the shop.

- ***It gives you total control of what you eat and the calorie intake.***

Advance food planning and preparation gives you total control of your keto diet, enabling the consumption of the right calories and keto macros balance. The chances of you eating foods that are not recommended or going above the recommended calories are closely managed or eliminated.

You know too well that controlling what you eat, the portion, and your calorie intake is important for dieting and weight loss. Keto meal prepping will keep you within the right measures and will help you to attain ketosis for a healthy, efficient body.

- ***It helps with hunger management.***

Hunger pangs are mainly triggered by predetermined mealtimes by habit. When the time comes when you normally eat dinner, you are likely to feel hungry. Keto meal prepping and planning will help you manage hunger by ensuring that you have the dish ready for the respective meal. Eating at the right time is also important to maintain the right ketosis metabolic balance.

- ***You get time to do other things.***

Whether you want to call it multitasking or getting time for other things, keto meal prepping will get that for you. The many hours you have from not cooking and preparing meals can be used for other activities, which will improve your performance and productivity in other areas of your life.

This is the ideal option for those with a busy life and tray that is always full. You want a meal plan in the first place because of the time factor. You are busy and would prefer getting more done within the often-short time that is available to you.

Even with the meal prepping process, you will be able to have multiple meals cooking because as something is baking in the oven, you could have another dish simmering on one burner, another stew on a different burner, and another burner frying another keto recipe, all within the prep time!

- ***It will bring variety to your meals.***

Keto meal prepping ensures that you have a variety of healthy foods every weekly cycle. By alternating products within every food category, you cannot get bored with what you eat because of the variety at your disposal. As we said, under the point of grocery shopping, you can eat different vegetables every day of the week or for every meal.

You will have the portions right, and the calorie intake will be as recommended. Consistency with the meals will help you to lose weight quickly.

Accordingly, this book is a great resource for those who are still looking into the keto diet and are considering whether it is the right diet for them to take up. You have the chance to learn about how keto meal prepping and planning works and how convenient it makes the dieting process for you.

Moreover, with all the benefits listed above, you will save time and money while still leading a healthy lifestyle and not compromising on your profession. In fact, you will have more time for your work and a healthy body to see you through the rigors of work.

For those on the keto diet and are not meal prepping and planning, this is another layer to the benefits you are already enjoying from the diet.

AN OVERVIEW OF STEPS TO GET READY FOR KETO MEAL PREPPING

Now that you know the benefits of a keto meal prep plan, we will have an overview of the steps and what you need to get ready for meal prepping. As much as there may be nuances in prepping the different meals, the general structure of getting ready for food prepping will remain the same throughout.

Here is what you need to do:

- **Step 1: Pick a day of the week.**

When you have enough time to outline a meal plan for the whole week.

Decide your meals by doing the following:

- Slot your picks in a calendar to correspond to the days and mealtimes.

- Go for ready recipes that have calories indicated and, if possible, macros listed so that you can easily adapt them to your preferences.

- Account for the number of people who will be served.

- Make it simple, having one meal more than once, either cooked or as a leftover.

- **Step 2: Map and plan the meals you have chosen.**

The next thing after picking out the meals you want for a week is to map out and plan the meals to meet keto nutritional requirements. Create different nutrition combinations for fat, carbohydrates, proteins, and vegetables. These combinations will help you with portioning the meals and drawing a supporting list of things to shop for.

- **Step 3: Make a shopping list, pick a shopping day, and shop for the ingredients.**

Write down the ingredients and other requirements, pick a convenient day to buy the items on your shopping list, and then shop for the items.

- **Step 4: Cook the keto meals.**

This is the final step in the prepping process. Once you have the ingredients ready, it is time to prep the meals and cook them accordingly.

QUICK START
ACTION STEP

For your meal prepping, follow the four steps above to cover all bases. Decide the keto diet meals you want and get the recipes, map, and plan the individual meals, make a detailed shopping list, and buy the required ingredients, and finally prep the ingredients and cook the meals.

In this chapter, we shall look at the things you need to have ready to begin meal prepping. We shall discuss the must-have kitchen equipment for meal prepping. We shall also look at how to stock your pantry with keto essentials and the type of storage containers you need for storing the meals you prepare.

GETTING READY FOR KETO MEAL PREPPING

When you have everything in place for meal prepping—the basic kitchen utensils and equipment, the meal prepping ingredients, and storage containers—you make meal prepping much easier. Preparing the pantry staples and kitchen equipment may seem time-consuming, but the opposite is true. It will save you time for the days and weeks to come.

Before you begin meal prepping, it would be wise to know the different ways of prepping meals, which will help with saving you time on the process so that you do not end up spending a whole day prepping your week's meals. The most popular ways to meal-prep include the following:

- Individual portions: Cooking fresh meals and portioning them into individual grab-and-go meals. Refrigerate and eat over the next few days. This is best for lunches.

- Ready-to-cook meals: This involves prepping ingredients for different meals in advance to save time when cooking.

- Cooking full meals in advance: You cook all the meals you want and refrigerate them. Warm them at mealtimes. This is convenient for dinners.

- Batch cooking: Cooking a large portion of one recipe and then dividing it into several portions, freezing them, and eating them for weeks or months. Best for lunches and dinners.

The method you choose for prepping your meals will be your preference and will probably be determined by your schedule and time management goals. Mixing different meal-prepping methods can also work depending on your unique circumstances.

The Benefits of Having Essentials Ready for Meal Prepping

Meal prepping can be challenging if you are a beginner, and you should, therefore, not be surprised or discouraged. It is very easy to get caught up in the nitty-gritty in trying to get it right. However, once you have the basics learned, you should take it easy and be practical. Do not try to do everything at once, and do not seek perfection. You should allow yourself room to wriggle and make mistakes from which you will learn from as time goes by.

Prepping meals is important for getting the keto diet right. Planning and prepping your meals ahead of time will help you stay within the recommended portions and nutritional counts.

Additionally, having the essentials of meal prepping ready—the equipment, ingredients, containers, and other requirements—may save you time in prepping and cooking. You will be stress-free and will get more done faster if you have things ready, having your meals for the week ready in no time and leaving the rest of the day to rest.

THE ESSENTIALS AND REQUIREMENTS FOR MEAL PREPPING

There are a number of kitchen equipment and tools that you must have to begin meal prepping. Additionally, you must have the essential ingredients for your recipes ready, as well as certain must-have keto diet ingredients. Having these kitchen tools and keto pantry staples is a time-saver.

The lists below have the essentials you should have ready for successful and stress-free meal prepping:

Kitchen Equipment and Tools

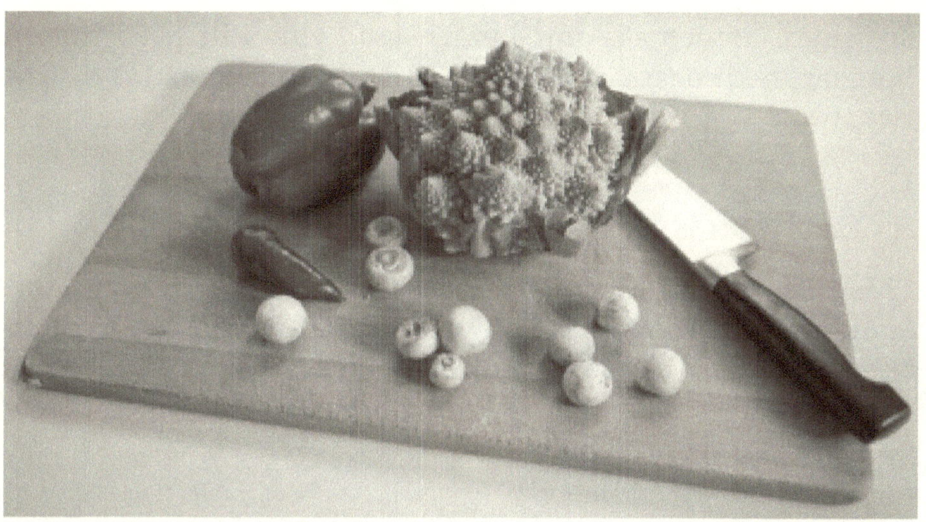

The following are some of the basic kitchen equipment and tools you need for prepping your keto-friendly meals. There are many household stores where you can get what you want at very affordable prices, as well as bargain sites like Amazon.

a. Skillet

A cast-iron skillet is a must-have in your kitchen for easy meal prepping, and it lasts a long time. It is easy to clean and offers better service than a pan.

b. Chef's knife

Since you will be doing a lot of dicing and slicing, you need a dependable knife that will serve you well for a long time. Getting a high-quality chef's knife will make cutting and slicing very easy.

c. Blender or food processor

The keto diet is full of meals and recipes that will require a blender or food processor. Certainly, for keto smoothies, salad dressings, homemade nut butter, etc., you will need one. A blender and processor in one is a good option instead of having two.

d. Instant Pot or pressure cooker or slow cooker

This is the perfect kitchen essential for slow and long cooking. Some of the keto recipes you will encounter will need you to cook broths and soups or slow cook meats, which require you to have a slow cooker. You will have other parts of a recipe slow cooking as you prep others.

e. Nonstick baking paper

Your keto oven meals and bakes will require nonstick oven paper.

f. Kitchen scale

You will need a kitchen scale to weigh some foods and ingredients. This is a perfect product for keto diet meal prep beginners who are just learning how to stay in ketosis.

There are so many kitchen tools that you can have to make your work easier in the kitchen. Here, we have only listed what we think are the essentials for you to have for keto meal prepping.

Stocking the Pantry with the Essentials

For the pantry, there are general cooking ingredients that you must have, and then there are keto essential ingredients that you will need to stock so that you do not miss a recipe item or make several time-wasting trips to the shop.

The following are what you should have for keto meal prepping:

1. Almond flour
2. Avocado oil
3. baking powder and baking soda
4. Butter (preferably grass-fed)
5. Celery salt
6. Cheese(s)
7. Cream cheese
8. Cinnamon
9. Cocoa powder
10. Coconut aminos
11. Coconut flour
12. Coconut oil
13. Eggs (free-range and pastured recommended)
14. full-fat coconut milk
15. Garlic cloves
16. Garlic powder
17. Ground beef (grass-fed recommended)
18. Heavy cream
19. Hot sauce
20. Keto sweeteners (erythritol, monk fruit, stevia, Swerve, Truvia)
21. Mayonnaise
22. MCT oil powder
23. Mustard (Dijon or yellow)
24. Nuts and seeds

25. Nut butters

26. Olive oil

27. Oregano

28. Parsley

29. Pumpkin pie spice

30. Red pepper flakes

31. Red wine vinegar

32. Sugar-free spices

33. Pepper and salt

34. Sour cream

35. Thyme

36. Unsweetened yogurt

37. Vanilla extract

38. high-fat oils

These are simply the essentials. You may stock as many as you want as long as they fit in the keto diet.

Storage Containers to Use

The containers you choose for storing your food storage can turn your food from a fabulous meal to an unenjoyable dish. Glass containers are the best for food storage because they are safe for microwave heating and warming. They do not have harmful chemicals as found in plastics.

In fact, use only glass containers for keto meal prepping, and make sure they are made for the microwave and oven.

Recommended Food Storage Container Specifications

- Airtight—to keep food fresh.

- BPA-free microwavable containers—go for Pyrex glassware.

- Compartmentalized containers—to enable you to have the different parts of a meal in one container.

- Freezer-safe containers—to limit freezer burn.

- Leak-proof

- Stackable—for better space management.

There are a lot of container options on the market for you to pick from. As long as they can be used in the oven or the microwave to heat or warm your food and meet the recommended food storage specifications above, the glass container will be good for use. You should also get them in different sizes so that you can pack different portions and recipes conveniently.

A high-quality food storage container should ensure that the nutrients in the food do not deteriorate quickly and that the food stays fresh and retains its taste.

QUICK START ACTION STEP

Now that you know the basics required of you to have before meal prepping, if you are a beginner, we would recommend shopping for the items you do not have a day before the actual meal prep, preferably when you will be shopping for recipe ingredients.

Meal planning and prepping is best on weekends when you are likely to have sufficient time to do it without distractions and disruptions. Saturday for shopping and Sunday for prepping works well.

This section will outline easy steps to guide you through successful keto meal prepping from beginning to end. You will mention the benefits of going by these steps and discuss each step of keto meal prepping in detail. Additionally, we will give you insights on how to calculate macros and why that is important.

HOW TO CALCULATE MACROS

We already know that for you to be successful with ketogenic dieting, you must plan every step and ensure that everything is done right. Calculating macros is one of the important aspects of ensuring success if you are on a keto diet.

To eat right, you need to pick the right keto recipes, which will require you to look at the calorie and macro contents of each meal and each day. Macros are the three main macronutrients of the keto diet, namely, fat, protein, and carbohydrates. While a regular diet is heavily reliant on carbs, the keto diet is fat-oriented.

You will need to eat foods with high quantities of fat, moderate protein, and very little carbs. It is easy when said; however, getting it right with every meal needs a keen tracking of the macro content.

The second option, specialized macro calculator, computes specific carb and protein targets, which you choose, thus not based on the classic keto ratios. There are several reasons why some people would want to do this.

It is important to note that this function is best left to those who have been on keto for some time, have achieved ketosis, and have a good understanding of how the diet works for them and interacts with their bodies.

When to use the standard keto calculation option:

- If you do not know your ketosis macros ratios.
- If you want exact ratios for every meal.
- If you are new to the ketogenic diet.
- If your reason for dieting is simply to lose, gain, or maintain weight.

When to use the specialized macronutrient calculation option:

- Pregnant or breastfeeding women who are measuring macros based on doctor advice.
- If you are adjusting macros ratios because of the keto rash.
- If your doctor recommends different macros ratios from the standard.
- If you have specific macro needs, e.g., an athlete.
- If you are on a high-protein keto diet.

The specialized macronutrient calculator should be used by those on keto who have special macros needs because of issues, like a very active lifestyle (athlete), a medical condition, or pregnancy.

How your bio details affect Your BMR:

- Age: BMR shrinks with age, starting after about thirty years, because of muscle mass decline.
- Gender: The body composition and performance of females and males differ.

- Height and weight: Needed to compute your unique body composition.

THE BENEFITS OF FOLLOWING THESE STEPS FOR KETO GOALS

The benefits of keto meal prep planning are probably what has got you interested in the keto diet in the first place or what led you to pick this book. The benefits of the steps here are the overall keto meal prepping and planning benefits, as discussed in detail earlier in chapter 1. Here is a quick recap of the advantages following these steps for meal prepping before we discuss the steps in detail.

The following is a list of the benefits of keto meal prep planning:

1. It saves time as compared to cooking daily.

2. Meal prepping is cheaper than cooking every day.

3. You do not decide what to eat every day.

4. You have better control of your food portions.

5. You have better calorie and macro-management.

6. Homemade food, especially by yourself, is delicious, healthier, and safer.

7. You have everything ready for cooking ahead of time.

Keto Meal Prep Planning Steps

1. *Plan the Meal Prep*

Planning entails picking a day for keto meal prepping, picking the meals you want for the week, and settling on the right recipes for the meals.

- *Pick the prepping day.*

The first thing to do is to pick the day for prepping the meals. Sunday is the best day because most people are off work and can enlist the help of others if you want. Some people opt for two days in a week to prep, which allows them to split meal prepping into two, usually Sunday and Wednesday.

- *Choose the meals.*

Once you have a day or have decided to split meal prepping into two days, choose the meals you want. Since we are focused on planning for a whole week, choose all the meals, desserts, and snacks that you want. Ensure that the meals are healthy and are keto compliant. You can also mark the meals on a calendar at this point.

- *Pick meal recipes.*

Once you know the meals you want, the next thing to do is to find keto recipes for the meals you have chosen. Keep the calories and macros in mind when picking the recipes so that you balance the meals correctly.

Beginners should choose easy recipes with a few ingredients. Even better, go for recipes that have similar ingredients—for instance, different meals with meats or vegetables—to make shopping and cooking easier.

Knowledge of how macronutrients are converted into calories will help you keep the right ratios. When choosing recipes, select the ones that you want to eat and will enjoy. It should not just be healthy; you should be happy about it.

- *Write down the week's keto menu.*

Once you have the recipes, write them down in the order you want to eat them during the week. Write down or print out the recipes so that you have them to follow on prep day. It also helps to craft the order in which the food is prepared. Start with the more engaging meals and finish up with the easy ones, like those for breakfast, desserts, and snacks.

- *Pick a prep day.*

This is the point where you decide if you want to do it on Saturday or Sunday or if you want to prep twice, say on Wednesday and Sunday. As advised earlier, it works best to prep a day after shopping, or you can choose to prep the same day you shop.

2. Write Down the Shopping List

Draw a shopping list of the ingredients from each of the recipes you have settled on. Break down the list into food categories—dairy, meat, vegetables, etc. The list must have the exact quantities of each ingredient as per the keto recipes. Avoid packaged and processed products.

Tip: Always check your fridge, freezer, and pantry to confirm what you have so that you do not overstock.

3. Go Shopping for the Items You Listed

Once you have the shopping list, all you have left is to buy what you need before you embark on the actual prepping. As said earlier, pick a convenient shopping day and time so that you are not drained by the experience. Shop when there is less traffic in the shops so that you will easily get what you want to leave.

Apart from the recipe items, buy the keto pantry essentials we listed earlier—any kitchen equipment and storage containers enough for the meals you will be preparing. Make sure you have your shopping list and stick to buying the items in it as planned.

4. Cook and Store the Meals

This is the point you have been preparing for—making the effort count and turning the recipes into delicious meals. Have all ingredients ready and the recipes out when doing this and follow them step by step.

Cooking can be tricky and may take longer than planned or suggested by the respective recipes, but keep going. It will be easier as you go along. Read through the recipes to understand what you need to do and how to do it. It is a good idea to start with those meals with the longest preparation process.

Those that need to be marinated or simmered for long periods should be dealt with first before the cooking day or hour so that everything is ready for the finalization of the dishes. All the veggies and meats that need to be prepared (cutting, slicing, dicing, marinating, etc.) should be done earlier so that they are ready on your cooking day. You may want to do this on shopping day after making your purchases or very early in the morning on prep day.

When packing the foods for storage, take into account the storage life of the various constituents of the meals packed, as well as recommended refrigeration times after cooking. For example, cut vegetables, like onions and peppers, will stay fresh under refrigeration for up to three days. Leafy vegetables, if dried, will last about a week, and cooked grains and meat dishes should be eaten within four days of cooking. Warm the meals at respective healthy temperatures when eating.

Tips:

- Newbies to keto and to meal prep should begin small and gradually prepare more meals once they learn and identify their favorite recipes and get a handle on meal prepping, respectively.

- When you start, choose simple recipes with a few ingredients and pick recipes with similar ingredients to shorten your shopping list and make cooking faster.

- If you are a beginner, you do not have to do a whole week. Try preparing three meals for starters to have a feel of the process.

- Start with some recipes that you have prepared before.

- Plan meals around seasonal produce for freshness and price value.

- Preparing the same dish for two or three mealtimes is a good energy-saving and time-saving idea for beginners.

QUICK START
ACTION STEP

Meal prepping is not a complicated process, is it? It may seem like at first, especially for a beginner, when you move from reading to actually doing.

Now what you need to do is to act on the steps learned here and follow through on the keto meal prep planning. Pick the meals you want and decide the meal prep day. Draw your shopping list to cover the ingredients, buy everything you need, and finally cook your meals and store them for the week ahead.

There is no better satisfaction than eating a delicious healthy meal prepared by yourself.

CHAPTER 6: WHAT IS A SLOW COOKER?

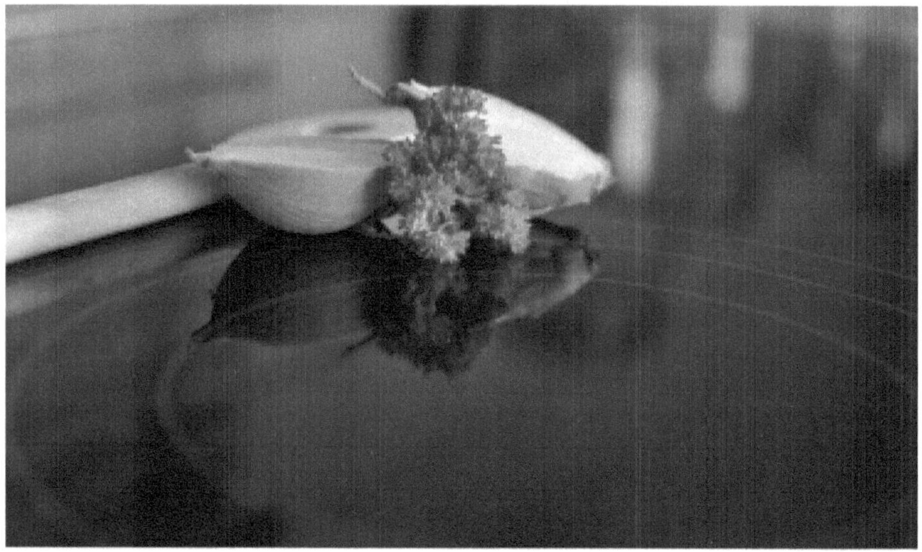

A Crockpot, also known as a slow cooker, is a countertop electrical equipment that is used to simmer or cook food at low temperatures. It is a multi-purpose kitchen appliance that allows you to cook soups, stews, pot roast, casseroles, and even desserts.

To use a Crockpot, take the raw food and liquid in the form of stock or water inside the Crockpot. Food is cooked at temperatures of between 700C and 800C. Because food isn't cooked at the boiling point, it retains more nutrients and enzymes as compared to when it's cooked conventionally.

The Crockpot comes with a heating component that keeps a steady temperature between 800C and 950C. The Crockpot comes with a lid that enables condensation inside the Crockpot. Also, the condensation from within the pot transmissions heats properly within the walls, so food is cooked all through.

ADVANTAGES OF CROCKPOT

Crockpots are very popular kitchen applications. They are heaven-sent to busy people as you can cook your foods while you are out so that they are ready by the time you are ready to eat. But more than suitability, there are also many aids to using Crockpots. Below are the advantages of using Crockpots when cooking your food.

- They are better at cooking inexpensive cuts of meat: Meats that come with connective tissues are cooked better in slow cookers. They can be stewed to create tastier dishware. By using Crockpots, you can make delightful meals without the need to buy costly cuts of meat.

- Food does not burn: Since food is cooked using low temperature, it does not burn even if it has been cooking for a long time.

- Brings out the full flavor of food: food cooked at low temperatures for a long time tends to have better flavor than those cooked in conventional cooking systems. Thus, if you are cooking casseroles, stews, soups, and one-pot meals, the

- Uses less electricity: A Crockpot does not consume too much electricity when cooking food so you can save on your electric bill even if it is running for a long time.

CHAPTER 7: MORNING RECIPES

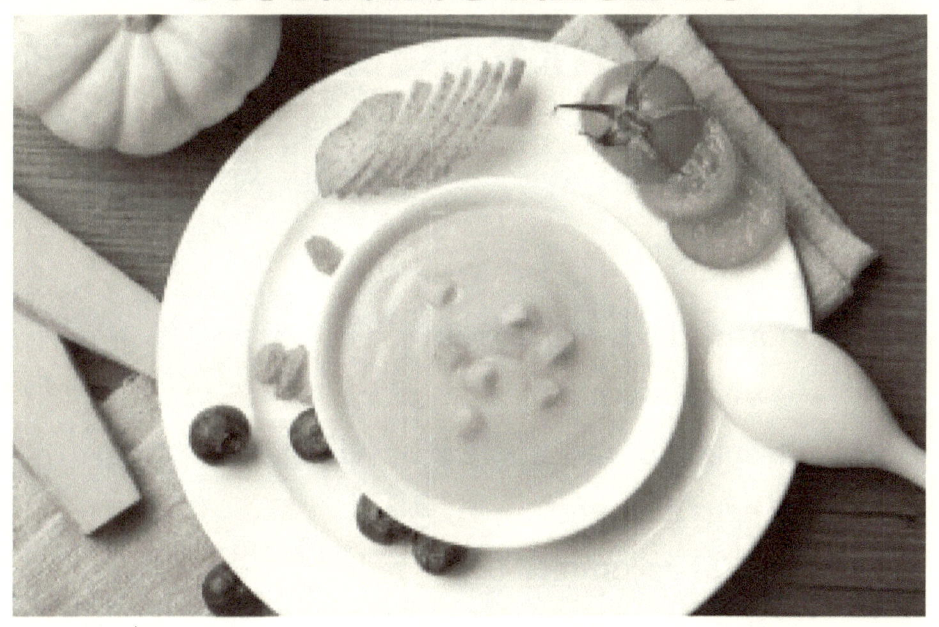

CROCKPOT PUMPKIN COCONUT BREAKFAST BARS

Preparation Time: 20 Minutes

Serves: 8

Ingredients:

- Canned puree pumpkin
- swerve sweetener
- a spoon of raw apple cider vinegar
- 3 eggs, beaten
- A c. of coconut flour
- Pumpkin pie spice
- Cinnamon
- Baking soda
- Salt
- 1/3 c. pecan, toasted and chopped

Directions:

1. Use a parchment paper lightly oiled with cooking oil.

2. Mix the pumpkin puree, sweetener, apple cider vinegar, and eggs.

3. Differently mix the salt, pumpkin pie spice, coconut flour, baking soda, and cinnamon.

4. Pour the wet ingredients to the dry ingredients and mix.

5. Pour the batter into the Crockpot and sprinkle with pecans.

6. Cover with lid. Cook for 3 hours on low or until a toothpick inserted in the middle comes out clean.

Nutrition information: Calories per serving: 187.4; Carbohydrates: 8.5g; Protein: 6g; Fat: 17.2g; Sugar: 2.5g; Sodium: 165mg; Fiber: 3g

OVERNIGHT EGGS BENEDICT CASSEROLE

Prep Time: 25 Minutes

Serves: 10

Ingredients:

- Canadian bacon, sliced
- 1 c. milk
- 10 large eggs, beaten
- 6 egg yolks
- Pepper and salt
- 2 tbsps. chives, chopped
- 1 ½ sticks butter, cubed

Directions:

1. Spray cooking oil in the Crockpot's ceramic interior.
2. Take the bacon slices at the bottom of the Crockpot.
3. Mix the eggs and milk. Season with pepper and salt.
4. Pour over the bacon.

5. Close the lid and cook for 1 ½ hours.

6. Open the lid and Take the egg yolks on top. Sprinkle with chopped chives.

7. Continue cooking for another 1 ½ hours or until the egg mixture is done.

8. While still warm, keep butter on top.

Nutrition information: Calories per serving: 256; Carbohydrates: 2g; Protein: 16.2g; Fat: 21g; Sugar: 0g; Sodium: 734mg; Fiber: 0.3g

CRUST-LESS CROCKPOT SPINACH QUICHE

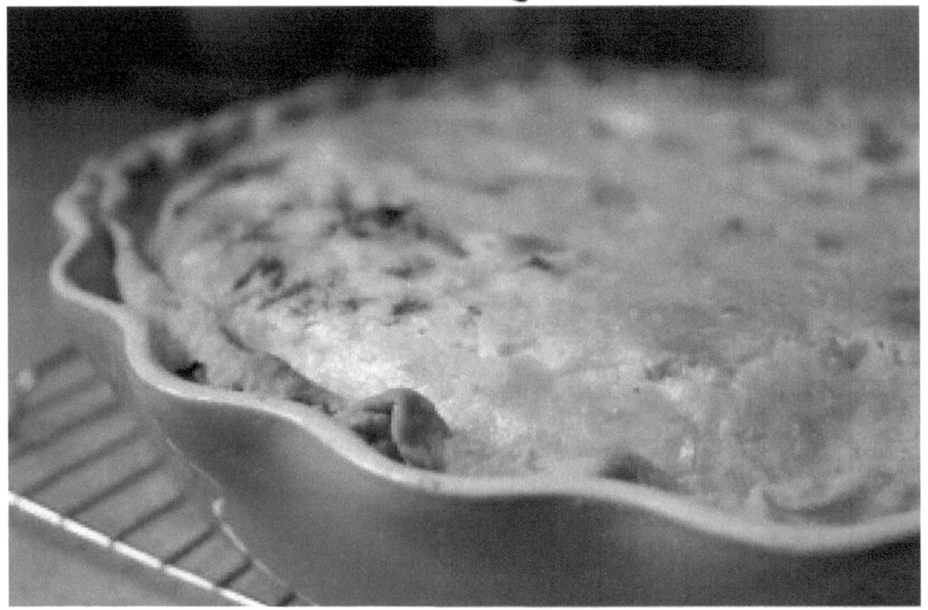

Prep Time: 50 Minutes

Serves: 6

Ingredients:

- Ghee

- 2 c. baby Bella mushrooms, chopped

- 1 medium red bell peppers, sliced

- 1 package chopped spinach, drained

- 8 eggs, beaten
- Sour cream
- Salt
- Black pepper
- Cheddar cheese, shredded
- 2 tbsps. chives, chopped
- Almond flour
- Baking soda

Directions:

1. Oil the slow cooker with cooking spray.

2. In a skillet, heat the ghee and sauté the mushrooms and bell peppers for 4 hours. Add the kale and cook for another minute.

3. Mix the eggs and sour cream. Season with pepper and salt. Stir in the cheese and chives. Add the almond flour and baking soda. Mix until well mixed. Stir in the vegetable mixture.

4. Pour the mixture in the Crockpot and cook on low heat for 5 hours or 3 hours on high heat.

Nutrition information: Calories per serving: 383.1; Carbohydrates: 7.3g; Protein: 15.1g; Fat:18g; Sugar: 0g; Sodium: 547mg; Fiber: 3.2g

CHEESY AND EGGY BREAKFAST CASSEROLE

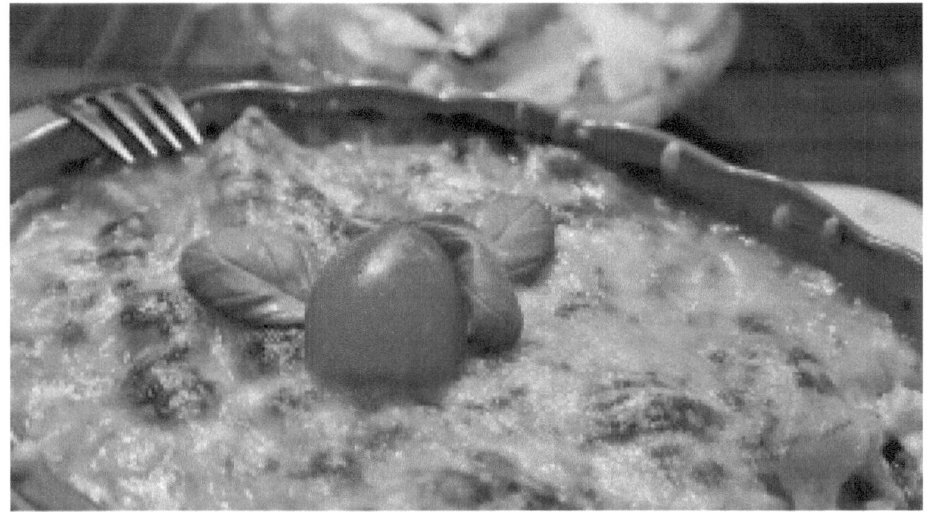

Preparation Time: 35 Minutes

Serves: 8

Ingredients:

- 12 eggs, beaten
- ¾ c. half-and-half
- Red pepper flakes
- Salt
- Ground black pepper
- Cheddar cheese, shredded

- 1 c. Colby cheese, shredded
- Green onions, chopped
- 1 cauliflower head, cut into florets
- 1-pound pork sausages, cooked and sliced
- ½ c. red bell peppers, roasted and chopped

Directions:

1. Line the sides of the cooker with foil. Oil with cooking spray.
2. mix the eggs, half-and-half, red pepper flakes, salt, and black pepper. Add the cheeses, onions, and cauliflower florets.
3. Take the sausages at the bottom of the Crockpot.
4. Pour over the egg mixture and top with chopped roasted bell peppers.
5. Close the lid and cook for 3 hours.

Nutrition information: Calories per serving:475; Carbohydrates: 5.2g; Protein: 23g; Fat: 26.7g; Sugar: 0.2g; Sodium: 791mg; Fiber: 2.1g

BROCCOLI AND TOMATOES CASSEROLE

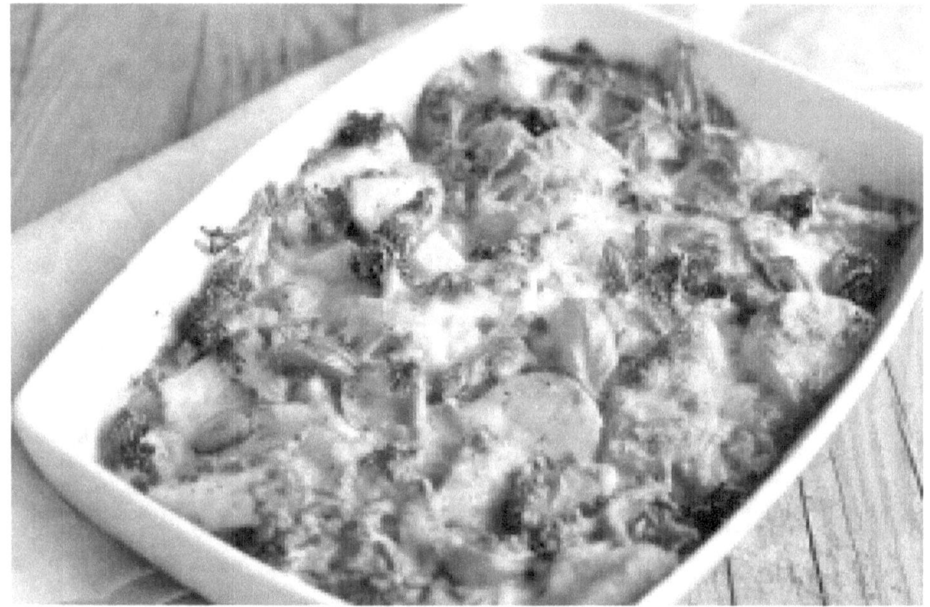

Prep Time: half an hour

Serves: 6

Ingredients:

- 1 large broccoli, chopped
- Butter
- Pepper and salt
- 1 ¼ c. cooked bacon, crumbled
- 1 ½ c. cherry tomatoes, halved

- 2 c. cheddar cheese, shredded
- 8 eggs, beaten
- ½ c. whole milk
- 1 bunch scallions, sliced

Directions:

1. Spray cooking spray on the interior of the Crock-pot.
2. Toss the broccoli and butter. Season with pepper and salt.
3. Press the vegetable mixture at the bottom of the Crockpot. Add the bacon and tomatoes on top. Add the cheddar cheese.
4. Mix the eggs and milk.
5. Pour the egg mixture over the vegetable layers. Sprinkle the scallions.
6. Close the lid and cook on low for 4 hours.

Nutrition information: Calories per serving: 486.; Carbohydrates: 8.1; Protein: 21.3g; Fat: 17g; Sugar: 2.9g; Sodium: 845mg; Fiber: 5.4g

SIMPLE HAM AND EGG CASSEROLE

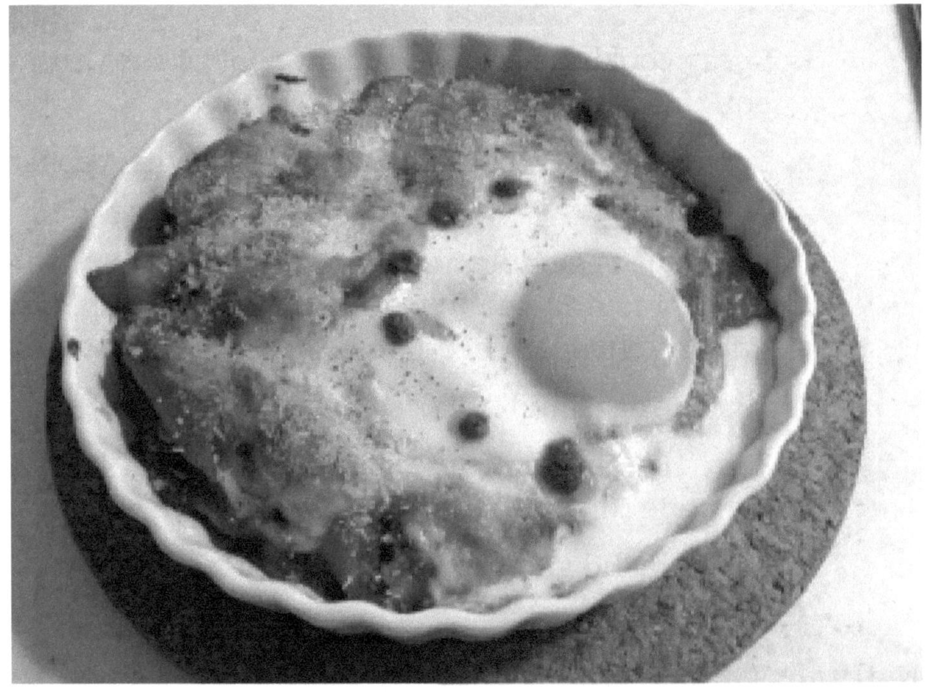

Preparation Time: 40 Minutes

Serves: 6

Ingredients:

- 4 tbsps. butter, melted
- ½ green bell pepper, diced

- ½ red bell pepper, diced
- 1 small onion, diced
- ½ c. ham, diced
- ½ c. cheese, shredded
- 6 eggs, beaten
- 1 tbsp. milk
- Pepper and salt to taste

Directions:

1. Spray the Crockpot with cooking spray.
2. Take melted butter in the Crockpot.
3. Add the bell peppers, onions, ham, and cheese in layers.
4. In a mixing bowl, mix the eggs and milk. Season with pepper and salt.
5. Pour over the layers of vegetables and ham.
6. Close the lid and cook for 3 hours on low or until a toothpick inserted in the middle comes out clean.

Nutrition information: Calories per serving:379.1; Carbohydrates: 7.2g; Protein: 15g; Fat: 20.4g; Sugar: 1.4g; Sodium: 744mg; Fiber: 3.9g

FLUFFY BREAKFAST OMELET

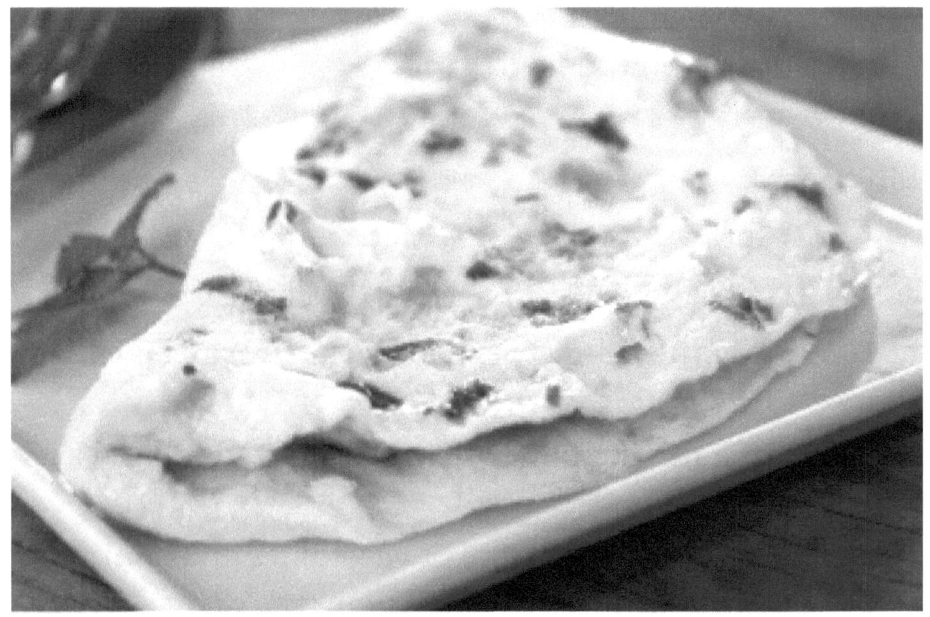

Preparation Time: 25 Minutes

Serves: 8

Ingredients:

- 4 strips bacon, cooked and crumbled
- 1 small onion, chopped
- 2 bell peppers, chopped
- 1 small head broccoli, chopped

- ½ c. cheddar cheese, shredded
- 4 egg whites
- 8 eggs, beaten
- ¾ c. milk
- 2 tsps. mustard, ground
- ½ tsp. garlic salt
- Pepper and salt to taste

Directions:

1. Oil the Crockpot with cooking spray.
2. Arrange in layers the bacon, onion, bell pepper, and broccoli.
3. Top with half of the cheddar cheese.
4. In a mixing bowl, beat the egg whites with a hand mixer until it forms stiff peaks. Set aside.
5. In another bowl, mix the eggs, milk, mustard, and garlic. Season with pepper and salt.
6. Fold the egg white mixture into the milk mixture gently.
7. Pour over the vegetable mixture.
8. Top with the remaining cheese.
9. Close the lid and cook for 3 hours or until a toothpick inserted in the middle comes out clean.

Nutrition information: Calories per serving: 320; Carbohydrates: 6.5g; Protein: 22.3g; Fat: 23.2g; Sugar: 1.9g; Sodium: 700mg; Fiber: 5.3g

CROCKPOT MEDITERRANEAN FRITTATA

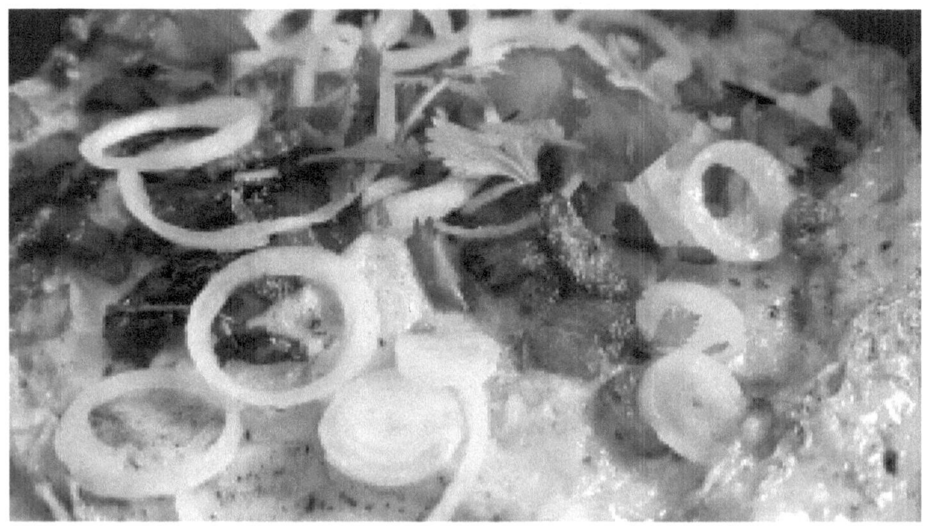

Preparation Time: 30 Minutes

Serves: 8

Ingredients:

- 8 eggs, beaten
- 1/3 c. milk
- 1 tsp. dried oregano
- Pepper and salt to taste

- 4 c. baby arugula rockets, rinsed and drained
- 1 ¼ c. red peppers, roasted and chopped
- ½ c. red onion, sliced thinly
- ¾ c. goat cheese, crumbled

Directions:

1. Spray cooking oil inside the Crockpot.
2. In a large bowl, mix the eggs, milk, and oregano. Season with pepper and salt.
3. Take the arugula leaves at the bottom of the Crockpot. Add the red peppers, onions, and goat cheese.
4. Pour over the egg mixture.
5. Cook on low for 3 hours.
6. Serve warm.

Nutrition information: Calories per serving: 416; Carbohydrates: 7.2g; Protein: 18.3g; Fat: 15.9g; Sugar: 1.3g; Sodium: 481mg; Fiber: 4.8g

SPINACH AND MOZZARELLA FRITTATA

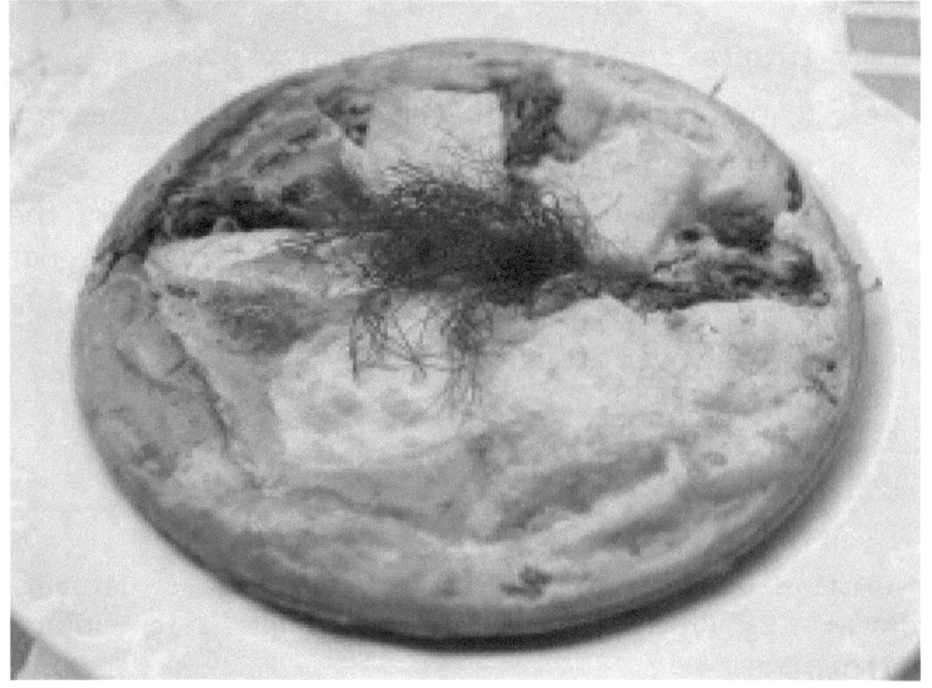

Preparation Time: 15 Minutes

Serves: 6

Ingredients:

- 1 tbsp. EVOO
- ½ c. onion, diced
- 3 eggs, beaten

- 1 c. mozzarella cheese, divided
- 2 tbsps. milk
- Pepper and salt to taste
- 3 egg whites, beaten until stiff peaks formed
- 1 c. baby spinach, rinsed
- 1 tomato, diced

Directions:

1. In a small skillet, heat oil and sauté the onions for 2 minutes. Set aside.
2. Spray the inside of the Crockpot with cooking spray.
3. In a bowl, mix the sautéed onions, eggs, mozzarella cheese, and milk. Season with pepper and salt to taste.
4. Fold the beaten egg whites to the egg mixture. Set aside.
5. Arrange the baby spinach and tomatoes at the bottom of the Crockpot.
6. Pour over the egg mixture.
7. Close the lid and cook for 3 hours on low or until a toothpick inserted in the middle comes out clean.

Nutrition information: Calories per serving: 139; Carbohydrates: 4g; Protein: 12g; Fat: 8g; Sugar: 2g; Sodium: 435mg; Fiber: 1g

ARTICHOKE HEARTS AND ROASTED PEPPER FRITTATA

Preparation Time: 30 Minutes

Serves: 8

Ingredients:

- 1 can artichoke hearts, drained and cut into small pieces
- 1 c. roasted red peppers, seeds removed and chopped
- ¼ c. green onions, sliced
- 8 eggs, beaten
- ½ c. feta cheese, crumbled
- Pepper and salt to taste
- Chopped parsley for garnish

Directions:

1. Take the artichoke hearts into the oiled Crockpot.

2. Add the red peppers and green onions.

3. In a bowl, mix the eggs and cheese. Season with pepper and salt to taste.

4. Pour over the vegetables.

5. Sprinkle parsley on top.

6. Cook on low for 2 ½ hours.

Nutrition information: Calories per serving: 322; Carbohydrates: 8.1g; Protein: 16g; Fat: 14.2g; Sugar: 0.6g; Sodium: 486.2mg; Fiber: 5.2g

SAUSAGE CAULIFLOWER BREAKFAST CASSEROLE

Preparation Time: 40 Minutes

Serves: 10

Ingredients:

- 1 head cauliflower, chopped finely
- 4 tbsp. unsalted butter, melted
- 2 tsps. salt
- 1-pound breakfast sausage
- 6 green onions, chopped
- 12 large eggs, beaten
- ½ c. mozzarella cheese, shredded

Directions:

1. Take the chopped cauliflower at the bottom of the Crockpot. Pour butter and season with salt.

2. Take the sausages and onions on top of the cauliflower bed. Pour over the beaten eggs and top with mozzarella cheese.

3. Cook on low for 3 hours.

Nutrition information: Calories per serving: 478; Carbohydrates: 5.7g; Protein: 16.3g; Fat: 22g; Sugar: 0.5g; Sodium: 550mg; Fiber: 3.8g

GREEK CROCKPOT BREAKFAST CASSEROLE

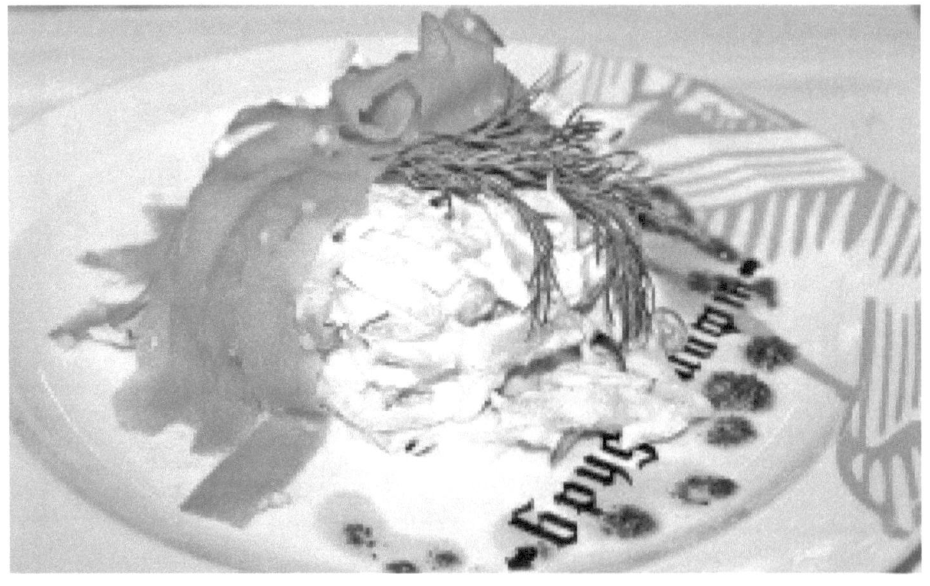

Preparation Time: 25 Minutes

Serves: 12

Ingredients:

- 12 eggs, beaten
- ½ c. milk
- ¼ tsp. black pepper
- ½ tsp. salt
- 1 tsp. garlic powder

- 1 tsp. onion powder
- ½ c. sun-dried tomatoes, soaked overnight
- ½ c. feta cheese, shredded
- 2 c. spinach
- 1 c. baby Bella mushrooms, sliced

Directions:

1. Lubricate the Crockpot with cooking spray.
2. Mix everything in a bowl.
3. Pour the mixture in the Crockpot.
4. Cook on low for 4 hours.

Nutrition information: Calories per serving: 397; Carbohydrates: 7.5g; Protein: 16.3g; Fat: 20.3g; Sugar: 1.2g; Sodium: 347mg; Fiber: 3.7 g

COCONUT CRANBERRY QUINOA PUDDING

Preparation Time: 40 Minutes

Serves: 10

Ingredients:

- ¼ c. dried cranberries
- 3 c. coconut water
- 1 tsp. vanilla extract
- 1 c. quinoa, uncooked
- 3 tsps. stevia extract
- 1/3 c. almonds, sliced
- 1/3 c. coconut flakes

Directions:

1. Take all ingredients inside the Crockpot.
2. Cook on low for 4 hours.
3. Serve warm.

Nutrition information: Calories per serving: 246; Carbohydrates: 4g; Protein: 8g; Fat: 5g; Sugar: 3g; Sodium: mg; Fiber: 5g

CROCKPOT BREAKFAST LETTUCE BURRITOS

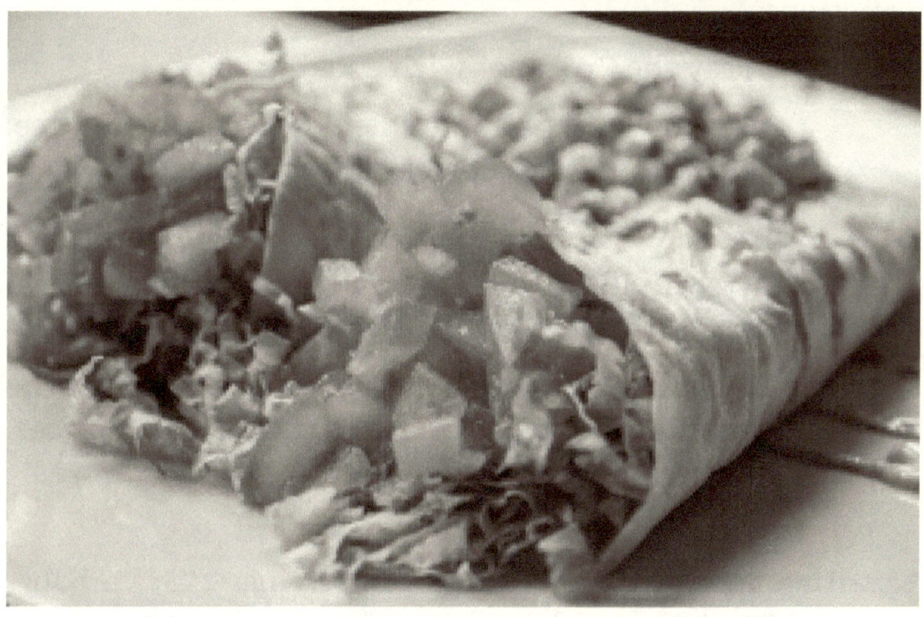

Preparation Time: 30 Minutes

Serves: 12

Ingredients:

- 12 eggs, beaten
- 1 c. milk
- 1 c. diced ham
- Pepper and salt to taste

- Lettuce leaves
- Cherry tomatoes, halved
- Chives, chopped
- Sour cream

Directions:

1. Spray the Crockpot with cooking spray.
2. In a bowl, mix all ingredients except the lettuce, cherry tomatoes, chives, and sour cream.
3. Cook on low for 4 hours.
4. After an hour, give the egg mixture a stir to create a scrambled egg-like consistency.
5. Bring together the lettuce burritos by placing the egg mixture on top of the lettuce. Add tomatoes, chives, and sour cream.

Nutrition information: Calories per serving: 275; Carbohydrates: 4.2g; Protein: 12.3g; Fat: 17.7g; Sugar: 1.2g; Sodium: 346mg; Fiber: 2.3g

BREAKFAST THREE CHEESE SHRIMPS

Preparation Time: 15 Minutes

Serves: 10

Ingredients:

- 6 c. chicken stock
- 1 tsp. dried thyme
- 1 tbsp. onion powder
- 1 tbsp. garlic powder
- Pepper and salt to taste
- 1 c. cheddar cheese, shredded
- 4 ounces light cream cheese
- ½ c. parmesan cheese, grated
- ½ tsp. hot sauce
- 2 pounds raw shrimp
- Chopped scallions for garnish

Directions:

1. Take all components except the scallions in the slow cooker.
2. Give a stir to incorporate everything.

3. Cook for 30 minutes or an hour on low.

4. Garnish with chopped scallions.

Nutrition information: Calories per serving: 472; Carbohydrates: 1.2g; Protein: 17.6g; Fat: 32g; Sugar: 0g; Sodium: 870mg; Fiber: 0.2g

CHAPTER 8: MIDDAY RECIPES

CROCKPOT BEEF ROAST

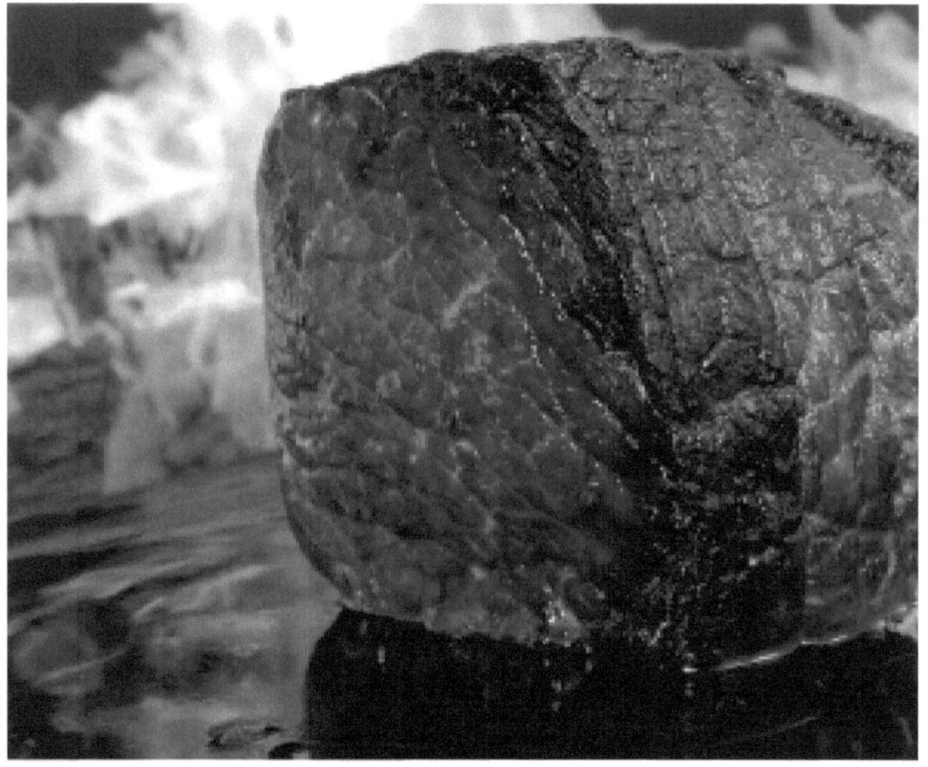

Preparation Time: 20 Minutes

Serves: 6

Ingredients:

- 2-pounds beef chuck roast, trimmed of excess fat
- 1 ½ tsps. salt
- ¾ tsp. black pepper

- 2 tbsps. fresh basil, chopped
- 4 cloves of garlic, minced
- 2 bay leaves
- 1 large yellow onion, chopped
- 2 c. beef stock

Directions:

1. Pat dry the beef roast with paper towel and rub with salt, pepper, and chopped basil.
2. Take inside the Crockpot and spread the onion, garlic, and bay leaves.
3. Pour over the beef stock.
4. Close the lid and cook on low for 10 hours until tender.

Nutrition information: Calories per serving: 234; Carbohydrates: 2.4g; Protein: 33.1g; Fat: 10.3g; Sugar: 0.9 g; Sodium: 758.2mg; Fiber: 0.5g

CHIPOTLE BARBECUE CHICKEN

Preparation Time: 20 Minutes

Serves: 5

Ingredients:

- ¼ c. water
- 1 14-ounce boneless chicken breasts, skin removed
- 1 14-ounce boneless chicken thighs, skin removed
- Pepper and salt to taste
- 2 tbsps. chipotle Tabasco sauce
- 1 c. tomato sauce
- 1/3 c. apple cider vinegar
- 1 onion, chopped
- 4 tbsps. unsalted butter
- 2 tbsps. yellow mustard
- ¼ tsp. garlic powder
- ½ c. water

Directions:

1. Take all ingredients in a Crockpot.

2. Give everything a stir so that the chicken is coated with the sauce.

3. Close the lid and cook on low for 8 hours.

Nutrition information: Calories per serving: 482; Carbohydrates: 3g; Protein:29.4 g; Fat: 18.7g; Sugar: 0g; Sodium: 462mg; Fiber: 0.3g

SPICY SHREDDED CHICKEN LETTUCE WRAPS

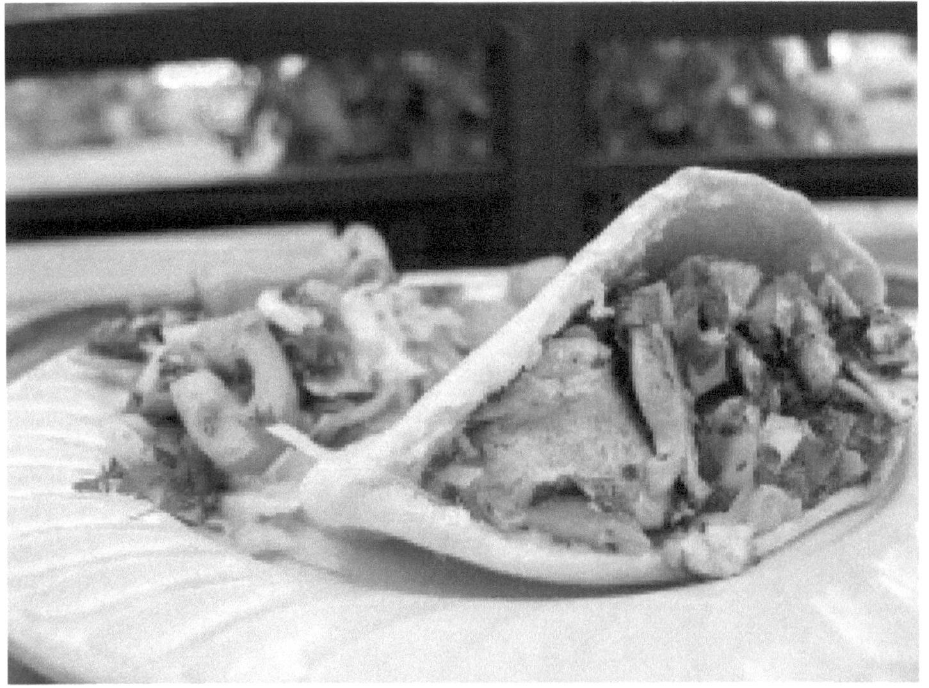

Preparation Time: 15 Minutes

Serves: 8

Ingredients:

- 4 chicken breast, skin and bones removed

- 1 c. tomato salsa
- 1 tsp. onion powder
- 1 can diced green chilies
- 1 tbsp. Tabasco sauce
- 2 tbsps. freshly squeezed lime juice
- Pepper and salt to taste
- 2 large heads iceberg lettuce, rinsed

Directions:

1. Take the chicken breast in the Crockpot.
2. Pour over the tomato salsa, onion powder, green chilies, Tabasco sauce, and lime juice. Season with pepper and salt to taste.
3. Close the lid and cook for 10 hours.
4. Shred the chicken meat using a fork.
5. Take on top of lettuce leaves.
6. Garnish with sour cream, tomatoes, or avocado slices if needed.

Nutrition information: Calories per serving: 231; Carbohydrates: 3g; Protein: 23 g; Fat: 12g; Sugar: 0.5g; Sodium: 375mg; Fiber: 2g

BACON CHEESEBURGER CASSEROLE

Preparation Time: 50 Minutes

Serves: 8

Ingredients:

- 2-pounds ground beef
- ½ onion, sliced thinly
- ½ tsp. salt
- ½ tsp. black pepper
- 1 15-ounce can cream of mushroom soup
- 1 15-ounce can cheddar cheese soup
- pounds bacon, cooked and crumbled
- 2 c. cheddar cheese, grated

Directions:

1. Brown the ground beef and onions in a skillet over medium heat. Season with pepper and salt to taste.

2. Take the beef in the Crockpot and add the cream of mushroom soup and cheese soup.

3. Pour in the bacon and half of the cheddar cheese. Give a stir.

4. Cook on low for 4 hours.

5. An hour before the cooking time is over, add the remaining cheese on top.

Nutrition information: Calories per serving: 322; Carbohydrates: 2g; Protein: 36g; Fat: 21g; Sugar: 0g; Sodium: 271mg; Fiber: 1.3g

CROCKPOT RANCH CHICKEN

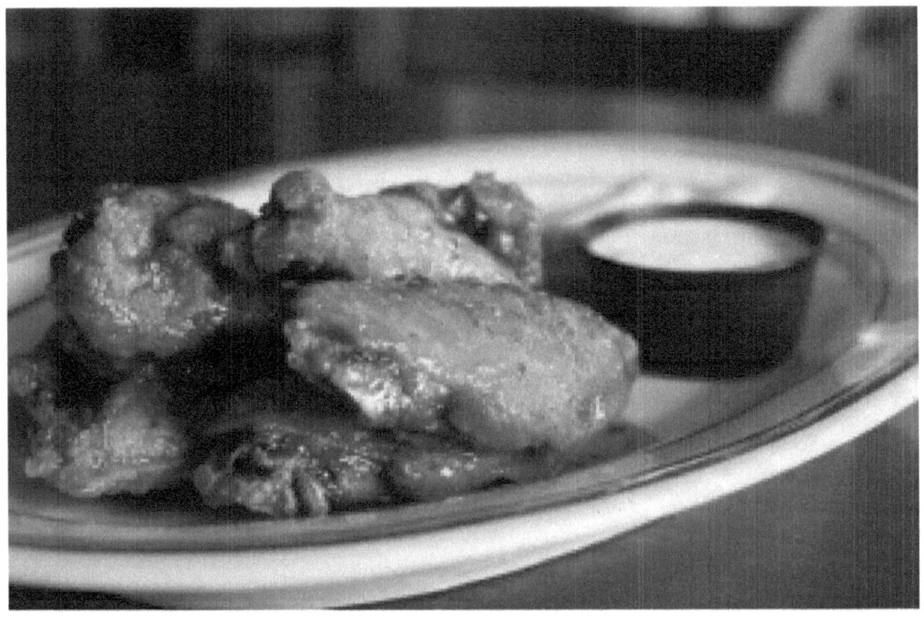

Preparation Time: 5 5 Minutes

Serves: 6

Ingredients:

- 2 pounds boneless chicken breasts
- 3 tbsps. dry ranch dressing mix
- 3 tbsps. butter
- 4 ounces cream cheese

Directions:

1. Take the chicken in the Crockpot. Pour the ranch dressing and rub on the chicken.

2. Add the butter and cream cheese.

3. Close the lid and cook for 7 hours on low.

4. Shred the chicken before serving.

Nutrition information: Calories per serving: 266; Carbohydrates: 0g; Protein: 33g; Fat:12.9g; Sugar: 0g; Sodium: 167mg; Fiber: 0g

COCONUT CILANTRO SHRIMP CURRY

Preparation Time: 40 Minutes

Serves: 4

Ingredients:

- 1 can light coconut milk
- 15-ounces water
- ½ c. Thai red curry sauce
- 2 ½ tsps. lemon juice
- 1 tsp. garlic powder
- ¼ c. cilantro
- Pepper and salt to taste
- 1-pound shrimps, heads removed only

Directions:

1. Take the coconut milk, water, and curry sauce in the Crockpot.

2. Stir in the lemon juice, garlic powder, and cilantro. Season with pepper and salt to taste.

3. Cook on high for 23 hours.

4. Add the shrimps and cook on high for 10

minutes.

Nutrition information: Calories per serving: 211; Carbohydrates: 2g; Protein: 18.2g; Fat: 22g; Sugar: 0g; Sodium: 135mg; Fiber: 0.8g

CROCKPOT BUTTER MASALA CHICKEN

Preparation Time: 45 Minutes

Serves: 8

Ingredients:

- 1 tbsp. olive oil
- 9 cloves of garlic, crushed
- 2 tsps. garam masala
- 2-pounds boneless chicken breasts, cut into strips
- 1 can light coconut milk
- 1 can tomato paste
- ½ tsp. cayenne pepper
- 1 tsp. dried coriander
- 1 tbsp. paprika
- 1 tsp. turmeric powder
- 1 tsp. cumin powder
- 1 ½ tsps. salt

Directions:

1. Heat olive oil in a skillet over medium flame and sauté the garlic for 1 minute. Add the garam ma-

sala and cook for another minute or until fragrant. Set aside.

2. Take the chicken in the Crockpot and add the garlic and garam masala mixture. Stir to coat the chicken meat.

3. Add the rest of the ingredients and cook on low for 7 hours.

Nutrition information: Calories per serving: 520; Carbohydrates: 2.3g; Protein: 32.7g; Fat: 28g; Sugar: 0g; Sodium: 342mg; Fiber: 0.8g

KASHMIRI LAMB CURRY

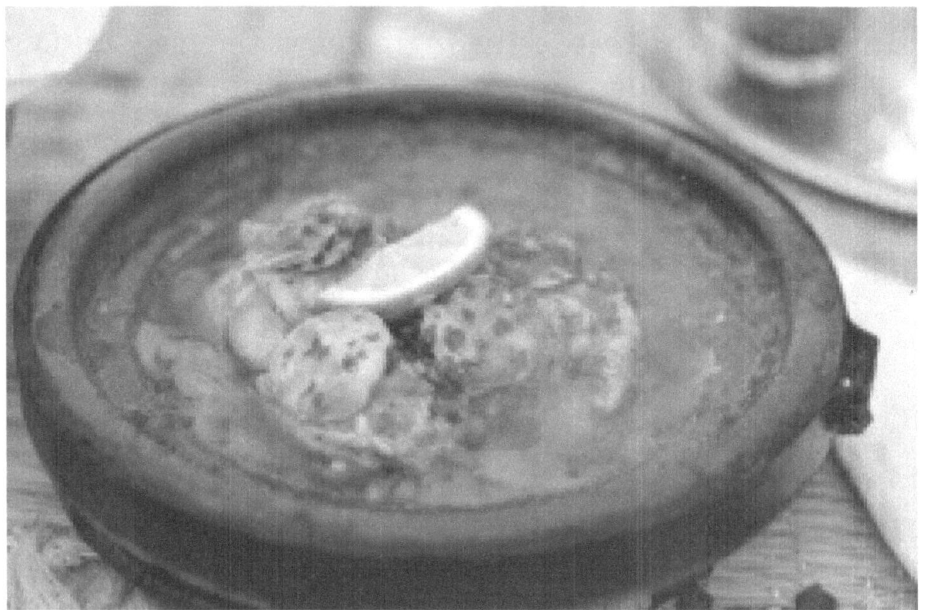

Preparation Time: 40 Minutes

Serves: 6

Ingredients:

- ¼ c. unsweetened coconut meat, shredded
- 3 long green fresh chili peppers
- 4 dried red chili peppers
- 1 tsp. garam masala
- 1 tsp. cumin seeds
- 5 cloves of garlic, crushed

- 1-piece ginger root, peeled and grated
- 2-pounds lamb meat
- 2 large onions, sliced
- 3 tomatoes, chopped
- 6 tbsps. vegetable oil
- ½ ground turmeric
- 1 c. plain yogurt
- ¼ c. cilantro, chopped
- 1 c. water
- Pepper and salt to taste

Directions:

1. Take the chilies, garam masala, cumin seeds, garlic, ginger, tomatoes, and coconut in a blender and pulse until smooth. Set aside.

2. In a skillet, heat vegetable oil and sauté the onions and lamb meat for 3 minutes.

3. Transfer the meat mixture in the Crockpot. Pour in chili paste mixture on top of the lamb.

4. Add the turmeric, yogurt, cilantro, and water. Season with pepper and salt.

5. Cook on low for 7 hours until tender.

Nutrition information: Calories per serving: 489; Carbohydrates: 3g; Protein: 25g; Fat: 40g; Sugar: 0g; Sodium: 166mg; Fiber: 2.5g

CHICKEN WITH BACON GRAVY

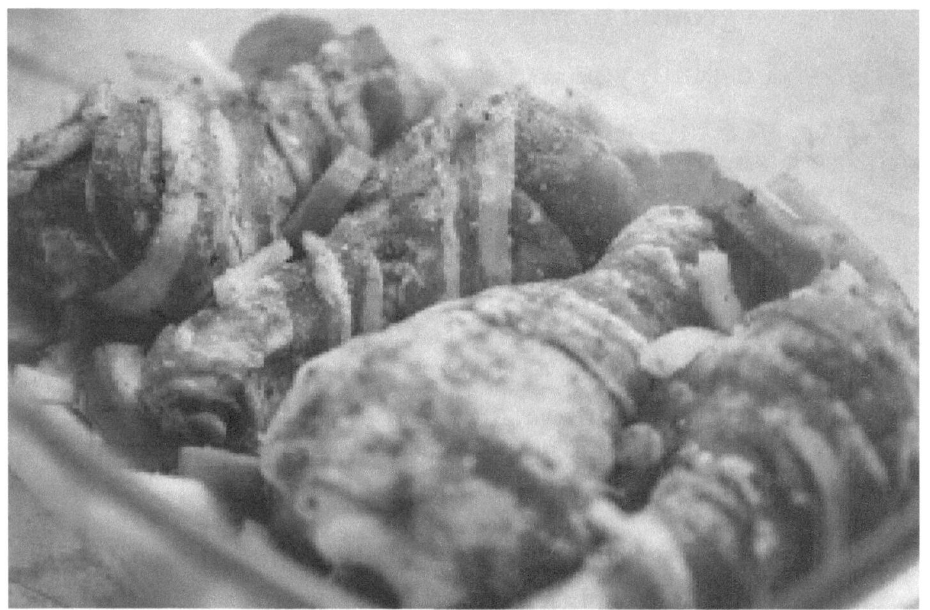

Preparation Time: 35 Minutes

Serves: 4

Ingredients:

- 1 ½ pounds chicken breasts, bones, and skin removed
- ¼ tsp. pepper
- 1 tsp. salt

- 1 tsp. minced garlic
- 1 tsp. dried thyme
- 6 slices of bacon, cooked and crumbled
- 1 ½ c. water
- 2/3 c. heavy cream

Directions:

1. Take all ingredients except the heavy cream in the Crockpot.
2. Close the lid and cook on low for 6 hours.
3. Add the heavy cream and continue cooking for another hour.

Nutrition information: Calories per serving: 359; Carbohydrates: 0.9g; Protein: 21g; Fat: 25g; Sugar: 0g; Sodium: mg; Fiber:0 g

GARLIC BUTTER CHICKEN WITH CREAM CHEESE

Preparation Time: 20 Minutes

Serves: 8

Ingredients:

- 2 ½ pounds chicken breast
- 1 stick of butter, softened
- 8 cloves of garlic, sliced in half
- 1 onion, sliced
- 1 ½ tsp. salt
- 8 ounces cream cheese
- 1 c. chicken stock

Directions:

1. Take the chicken in the Crockpot and add the butter.
2. Stir in the garlic and onions. Season with salt.
3. Cook on low for 6 hours.
4. Meanwhile, prepare the cream cheese sauce by mixing together cream cheese and chicken stock

in a saucepan. Heat over medium flame and stir until the sauce has reduced.

5. Pour over the chicken.

Nutrition information: Calories per serving: 463; Carbohydrates:2 g; Protein: 22.4g; Fat: 35g; Sugar: 0g; Sodium: 674mg; Fiber: 0.6g

CHEESY ADOBO CHICKEN

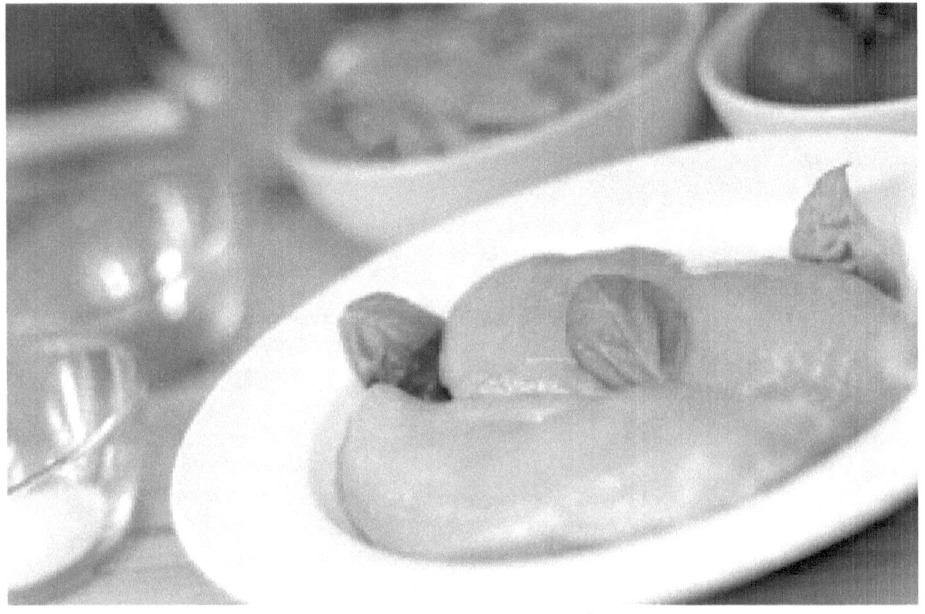

Preparation Time: 30 Minutes

Serves: 6

Ingredients:

- 1 pound of chicken breasts, bones removed but skin on
- 1 tbsp. butter
- ½ c. tomatoes, sliced

- 2 tbsps. adobo sauce
- ½ c. milk
- ¾ c. cheddar cheese, shredded

Directions:

1. Take all ingredients in the Crockpot.
2. Give a stir and cook on low for 8 hours.
3. Use a fork to shred the chicken.

Nutrition information: Calories per serving: 493; Carbohydrates: 0g; Protein: 25.8g; Fat: 33.9g; Sugar: 0g; Sodium: 375mg; Fiber: 0g

KETOGENIC CHICKEN TIKKA MASALA

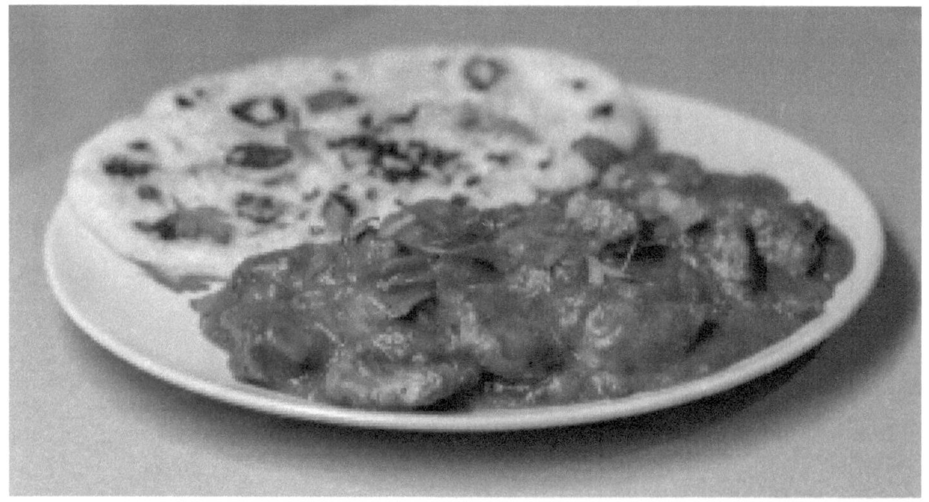

Preparation Time: 25 Minutes

Serves: 6

Ingredients:

- **1 ½ pounds chicken thighs, bone-in, and skin-on**
- **2 tsps. onion powder**
- **2 tbsps. olive oil**
- **5 tsps. garam masala**
- **3 tbsps. tomato paste**

- **1-inch ginger root, grated**
- **3 cloves of garlic**
- **2 tsps. smoked paprika**
- **1 c. heavy cream**
- **1 c. tomatoes, diced**
- **1 c. coconut milk**
- Salt to taste
- Fresh cilantro for garnish

Directions:

1. Take all ingredients except the cilantro in the Crockpot.
2. Mix everything until the spices are incorporated well.
3. Close the lid and cook on low for 8 hours.
4. Garnish with cilantro once cooked.

Nutrition information: Calories per serving: 493; Carbohydrates:4.3g; Protein: 26.6g; Fat: 41.2g; Sugar: 1g; Sodium: 457mg; Fiber: 2g

BALSAMIC CHICKEN THIGHS

Preparation Time: 30 Minutes

Serves: 8

Ingredients:

- 1 tsp. dried basil
- 2 tsps. minced onion
- 1 tsp. garlic powder
- ½ tsp. salt
- ½ tsp. black pepper
- 8 boneless chicken breasts
- 1 tbsp. EVOO
- 4 cloves of garlic, minced
- ½ c. balsamic vinegar
- Parsley for garnish

Directions:

1. In a small bowl, mix the dried basil, onion, garlic, salt, and pepper.

2. Rub the spice mixture onto the chicken. Set aside

3. Take olive oil in the Crockpot and sprinkle minced garlic.

4. Arrange the chicken piece on top of the oil and garlic

5. Pour balsamic vinegar.

6. Cook on low for 8 hours.

7. Garnish with parsley once cooked.

Nutrition information: Calories per serving: 133; Carbohydrates: 5.6g; Protein: 20.1g; Fat: 4g; Sugar: 3g; Sodium: 832mg; Fiber: 0.1g

CHICKEN LO MEIN

Preparation Time: 40 Minutes

Serves: 6

Ingredients:

- 1 ½ pounds chicken, sliced into strip
- 1 tbsp. coconut aminos
- ½ tsp. sesame oil
- ½ tsp. garlic paste
- 2 cloves of garlic, minced
- 1 tsp. ginger, minced
- bunch bok choy, washed and sliced
- 12 ounces kelp noodles
- Pepper and salt to taste
- ¾ c. chicken broth
- 1 tbsp. rice vinegar
- 1 tsp. red pepper chili flakes

Directions:

1. In a small bowl, mix the chicken, coconut aminos, sesame oil, and garlic paste. Let it marinate for 30 minutes inside the fridge.

2. Cook the marinated chicken in the Crockpot on high for 2 hours. Set aside.

3. Take the garlic, ginger, and bok choy at the bottom of the Crockpot. Add the chicken and kelp noodles on top. Season with pepper and salt to taste.

4. In a bowl, mix the chicken broth, rice vinegar, and red pepper flakes.

5. Pour over the chicken mixture and cook for 30 minutes on high.

Nutrition information: Calories per serving: 174; Carbohydrates: 3.1g; Protein: 24.5g; Fat: 8.1g; Sugar: 0.5g; Sodium: 436mg; Fiber: 1.6g

ETHIOPIAN DORO WATT CHICKEN

Preparation Time: 35 Minutes

Serves: 6

Ingredients:

- 1 tsp. chili powder
- 1 tsp. sweet paprika
- ½ tsp. ground ginger
- 1 tbsp. salt
- 1 tsp. ground coriander
- 1/8 tsp. ground cardamom
- 1/8 tsp. allspice
- 1/8 tsp. fenugreek powder
- 1/8 tsp. nutmeg
- 1 whole chicken, sliced into different parts
- ½ c. butter
- 1 clove of garlic, minced
- 1/2 c. water
- 2 large onions, chopped
- 8 hard-boiled eggs

Directions:

1. Mix the first 9 ingredients in a bowl. Use this spice mix and rub it on the chicken parts. Let the chicken marinate for 30 minutes in the fridge.

2. Take the butter in the Crockpot and add the onion and garlic. Take the chicken pieces. Arrange the hardboiled eggs randomly on top of the chicken.

3. Pour water.

4. Close the lid and cook on low for 8 hours.

Nutrition information: Calories per serving: 315; Carbohydrates:4g; Protein: 19g; Fat: 25g; Sugar: 0g; Sodium: 698mg; Fiber: 0.8g

CHAPTER 9: RECIPES FOR DINNER

BACON CHEDDAR BROCCOLI SALAD

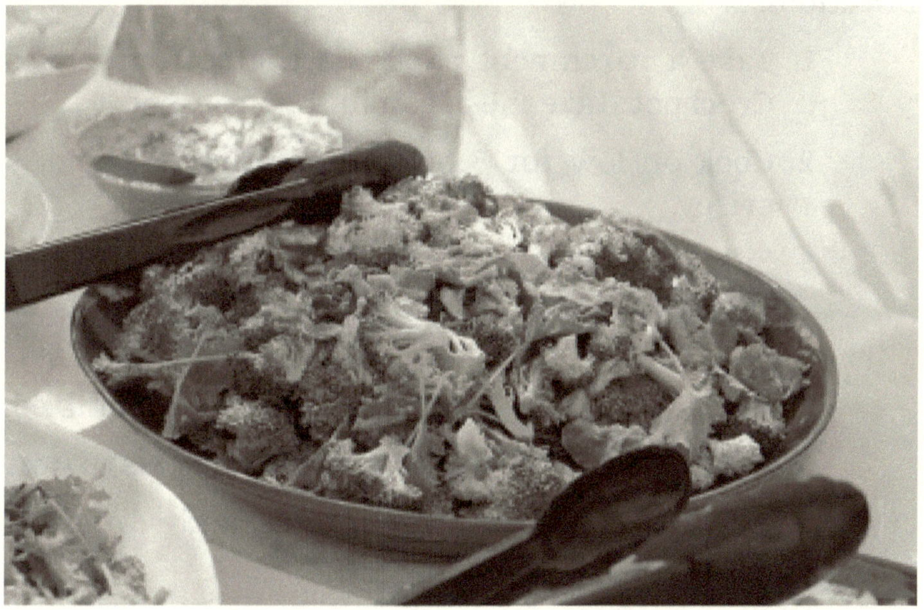

Preparation Time: 35 Minutes

Serves: 6

Ingredients:

- 6 slices raw bacon, chopped
- 1 bunch steamed broccoli, cut into small florets
- ¾ c. mayonnaise
- 2 tbsps. apple cider vinegar

- 3 packets stevia powder
- ½ c. cheddar cheese
- ¼ c. onion, chopped
- ¼ c. sunflower seeds, roasted

Directions:

1. Take a parchment paper on the bottom of the Crockpot. Take the bacon in the Crockpot.
2. Cook on low for 8 hours or until the bacon is crispy.
3. Take the bacon in a bowl and add the steamed broccoli.
4. In another bowl, add the mayonnaise, apple cider vinegar, and stevia powder. Mix until well mixed.
5. Pour over the bacon and broccoli and toss to mix.
6. Add the cheddar cheese, onion, and sunflower seeds.

Nutrition information: Calories per serving: 231; Carbohydrates:8.1 g; Protein: 16g; Fat: 15.3g; Sugar: 2.4g; Sodium: 751mg; Fiber: 3g

CHICKEN YELLOW CURRY

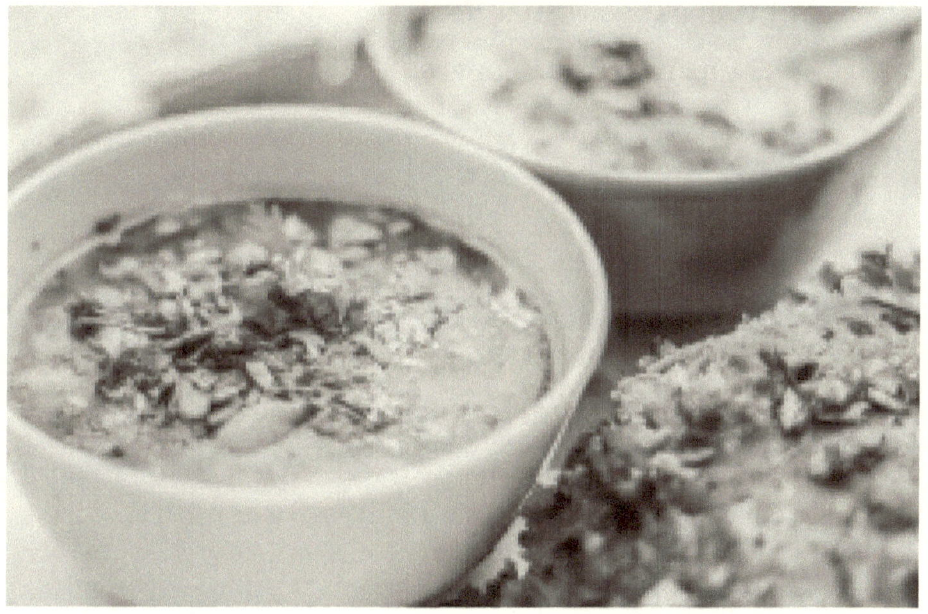

Preparation Time: 40 Minutes

Serves: 6

Ingredients:

- 1 ½ pounds chicken breasts, skin and bones re-moved
- 6 c. mixed vegetables (preferably broccoli, and cauliflower)
- 1 can full-fat coconut milk

- 2 tsps. ground ginger
- 1 tsp. cinnamon
- 1 c. water
- 2 tsps. ground coriander
- 2 tsps. ground ginger powder
- 1 c. crushed tomatoes
- ½ tsp. cayenne pepper
- 1 tbsp. cumin
- Salt to taste

Directions:

1. Take the chicken and vegetables in the Crockpot.
2. Add the rest of the ingredients and stir to mix everything.
3. Close the lid and cook on low for 6 hours.

Nutrition information: Calories per serving: 425; Carbohydrates: 3g; Protein: 23g; Fat: 31.4g; Sugar: 0g; Sodium: 371.4mg; Fiber:0.9 g

THAI WHOLE CHICKEN SOUP

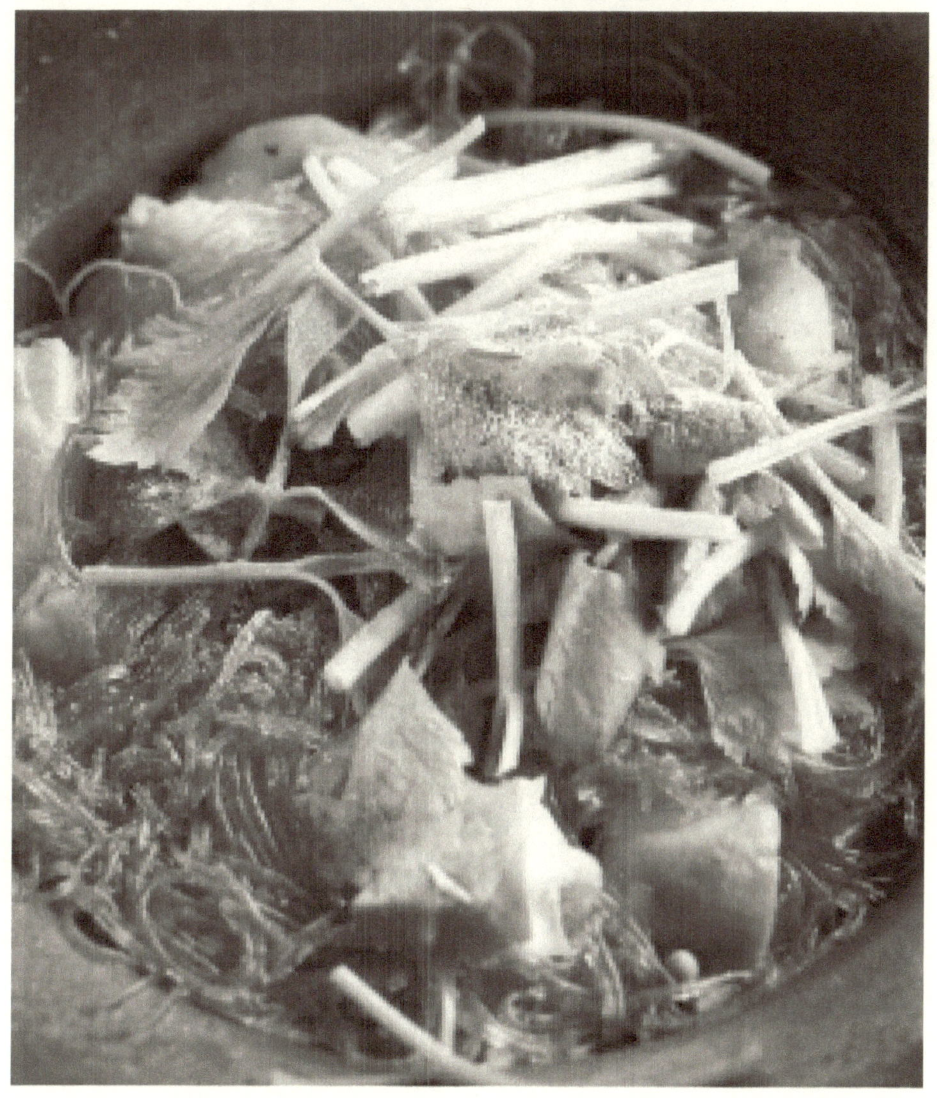

Preparation Time: 25 Minutes

Serves: 10

Ingredients:

- 1 whole chicken
- 1 stalk lemongrass, cut into chunks
- 20 fresh basil leaves
- 5 thick slices of ginger
- 1 tbsp. salt or more if needed
- 1 lime, sliced

Directions:

1. Take the whole chicken inside the Crockpot.
2. Surround it with lemongrass stalks, 10 basil leaves, and ginger.
3. Fill the Crockpot with water until the maximum line. Season with salt.
4. Cook on low for 10 hours or until the chicken is tender.
5. Serve with lime and the remaining basil leaves.

Nutrition information: Calories per serving: 475; Carbohydrates: 2g; Protein: 42g; Fat: 12g; Sugar: 0g; Sodium: 278mg; Fiber:0.5g

LEMON GRASS AND COCONUT CHICKEN DRUMSTICKS

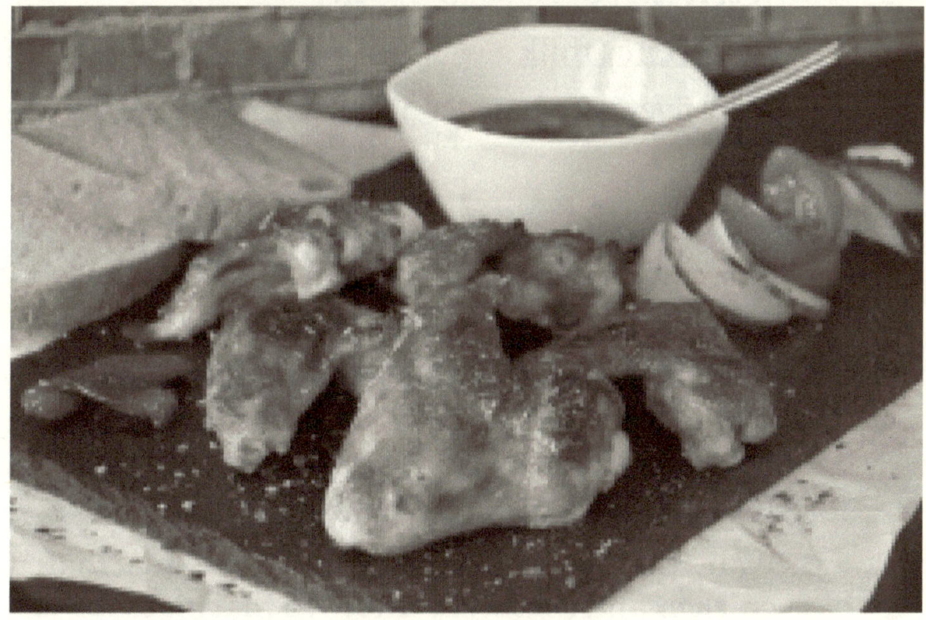

Preparation Time: 15 Minutes

Serves: 6

Ingredients:

- 10 drumsticks, skin removed

- Pepper and salt to taste

- 1 stalk lemongrass, cut into 5-inches long sticks

- 3 tbsps. coconut aminos
- 3 tbsp. EVOO
- 1 thumb-size ginger
- 1 large onion, sliced thinly
- 4 cloves of garlic, minced
- 2 tbsps. fish sauce
- ¼ c. fresh scallions, chopped
- 1 c. coconut milk
- 1 tsp. five-spice powder

Directions:

1. Take the chicken drumstick in a bowl and season with pepper and salt. Set aside.

2. In a blender, take the lemongrass, oil ginger, garlic, fish sauce, coconut milk, aminos, and five-spice powder. Blend until a smooth paste is formed.

3. Pour the paste or sauce into the marinated chicken and mix well. Allow to marinate for another 2 hours.

4. Take the onion in the Crockpot and add the marinated chicken.

5. Cook on low for 8 hours.

6. Sprinkle with scallions on top.

Nutrition information: Calories per serving: 528; Carbohydrates: 2g; Protein: 32g; Fat: 27g; Sugar: 0g; Sodium: 325mg;

Fiber: 0.8g

CROCKPOT BEEF STROGANOFF

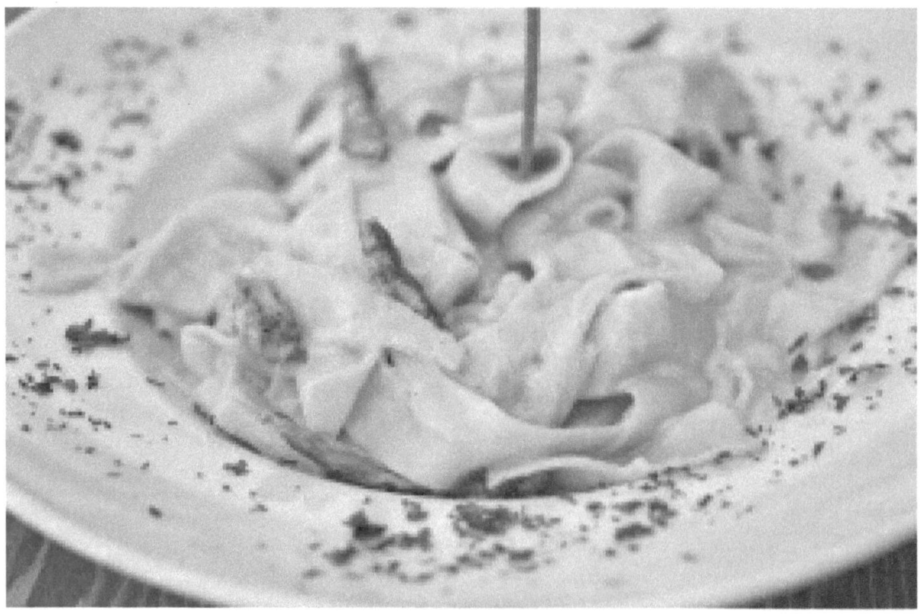

Preparation Time: 30 Minutes

Serves: 8

Ingredients:

- 2-pounds beef stew meat
- 2 tsps. salt
- ½ tsp. black pepper
- 1 tsp. garlic powder

- 3 tbsps. EVOO
- 2 tsps. paprika
- 1 tsp. thyme
- 1 tsp. onion powder
- 8 ounces mushrooms, sliced
- 1 small onion, sliced
- 1/3 c. coconut cream
- 2 tsps. vinegar

Directions:

1. Season the beef stew meat with pepper and salt. Add the garlic powder, oil, paprika, thyme, and onion powder. Stir to mix all ingredients. Let the beef marinate for 2 hours inside the fridge.

2. Take the mushrooms and onion in the Crockpot and Take the seasoned beef on top.

3. Close the lid and cook on low for 8 hours.

4. Once the meat is nearly done, add the coconut cream and vinegar. Adjust the seasoning if needed.

Nutrition information: Calories per serving: 381; Carbohydrates:2 g; Protein: 27.9g; Fat:24.5 g; Sugar: 0g; Sodium: mg; Fiber:0.9 g

SPAGHETTI SQUASH WITH SHRIMP SCAMPI

Preparation Time: 30 Minutes

Serves: 4

Ingredients:

- 2 c. chicken broth
- 1 small onion, chopped
- 2 ½ tsp. lemon-garlic seasoning
- 1 tbsp. butter or ghee
- 3 pounds spaghetti squash, cut crosswise and seeds removed
- ¾ pounds shrimp, shelled and deveined
- Pepper and salt to taste.

Directions:

1. Pour broth in the Crockpot and stir in the lemon garlic seasoning, onion, and butter.

2. Take the spaghetti squash and cook on high for hours.

3. Once cooked, remove the spaghetti squash from the Crockpot and run a fork through the meat to create the strands.

4. Take the squash strands back to the Crockpot and add the shrimps.

5. Season with pepper and salt.

6. Continue cooking on high for 30 minutes or until the shrimps have turned pink.

Nutrition information: Calories per serving: 363.3; Carbohydrates:1 g; Protein: 33g; Fat:21.2g; Sugar: 0g; Sodium: 276.2mg; Fiber:0.1 g

CROCKPOT GARLIC AND SHRIMPS

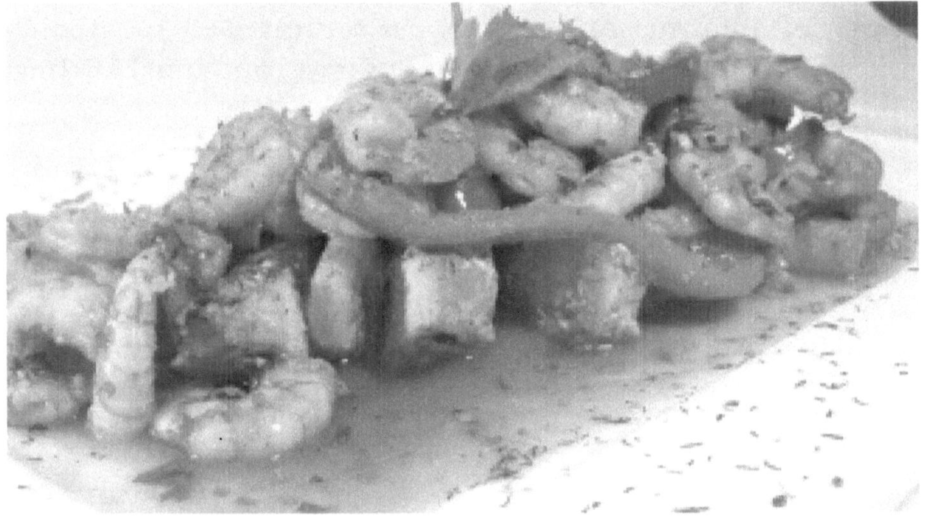

Preparation Time: 20 Minutes

Serves: 10

Ingredients:

- ¾ c. extra virgin olive oil
- 6 cloves of garlic, sliced
- 1 tsp. smoked Spanish paprika
- 1 tsp. salt
- ¼ tsp. black pepper
- ¼ tsp. red pepper flakes, crushed

- 2-pounds raw shrimp, shells removed and de-veined

- 1 tbsp. parsley, minced

Directions:

1. In a small bowl, mix together olive oil, garlic, paprika, salt, pepper, and red pepper flakes.

2. Take the shrimp in the Crockpot and pour the spice mixture.

3. Stir to mix all ingredients.

4. Cook on low for 1 hour.

5. Garnish with parsley.

Nutrition information: Calories per serving: 429; Carbohydrates:1 g; Protein: 18g; Fat: 24.5g; Sugar: 0g; Sodium: 211mg; Fiber: 0g

PORK STEW WITH OYSTER MUSHROOMS

Preparation Time: 25 Minutes

Serves: 4

Ingredients:

- 2 tbsp. coconut oil
- medium onion, chopped
- 1 clove of garlic, chopped
- 2 pounds pork loin, cut into cubes
- Pepper and salt to taste
- 2 tbsps. oregano
- 2 tbsps. dried mustard
- ½ tsp. ground nutmeg
- 1 ½ c. bone broth
- 2 pounds oyster mushroom, rinsed
- ¼ c. full fat coconut milk
- ¼ c. ghee
- 3 tbsp. capers

Directions:

1. In a skillet, melt the coconut oil over medium

flame. Sauté the onion and garlic until fragrant. Add the pork loin and brown all sides. Season with pepper and salt to taste.

2. Transfer the sautéed meat, garlic, and onions in the Crockpot.

3. Add the oregano, mustard, nutmeg, bone broth, and oyster mushrooms.

4. Give a stir and cook on low for 10 hours.

5. Before the meat is nearly cooked, add the coconut milk and ghee.

6. Once done cooking, garnish with capers.

Nutrition information: Calories per serving: 734; Carbohydrates: 12.5g; Protein: 50.4g; Fat:48.9g; Sugar: 2.3g; Sodium: 1118mg; Fiber: 7.9g

EASY CROCKPOT PORK LOIN

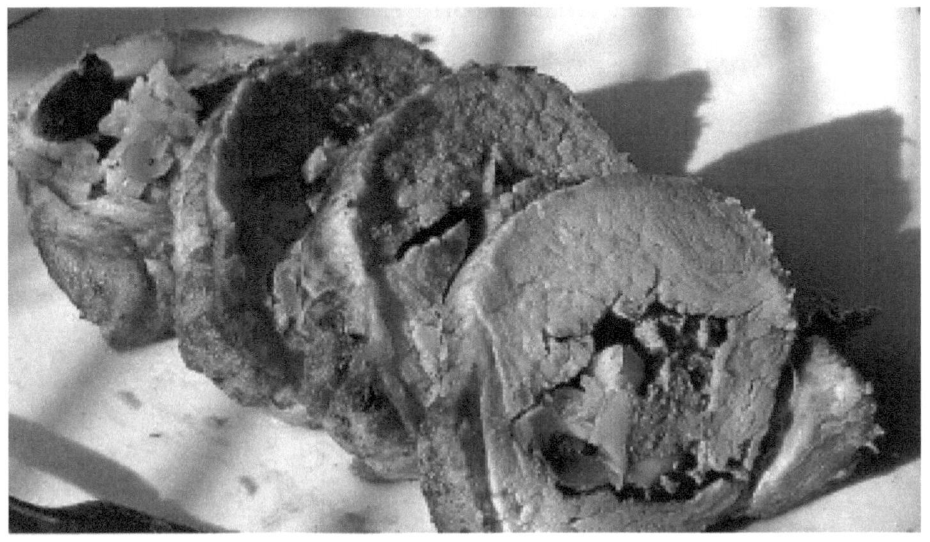

Preparation Time: 40 Minutes

Serves: 12

Ingredients:

- 5 pounds pork loin
- Pepper and salt to taste
- 2 onions, chopped
- 3 c. beef broth

Directions:

1. Season the pork loin with pepper and salt.

2. Take inside the Crockpot and arrange the onions around the roast.

3. Pour the beef broth.

4. Cook on low for 10 hours until tender.

Nutrition information: Calories per serving: 372; Carbohydrates: 0g; Protein: 37.5g; Fat: 23.4g; Sugar: 0g; Sodium: 261mg; Fiber: 0g

STICKY CHICKEN WINGS

Preparation Time: 20 Minutes

Serves: 6

Ingredients:

- ¼ tsp. salt
- 2 tbsps. Chinese five-spice powder
- 3 tbsps. coconut aminos
- 1 tsp. sesame oil
- ¾ tsp. red pepper flakes
- 1 tbsp. ginger, minced
- 2 tbsps. garlic, minced
- 1 tbsp. xanthan gum
- 3 pounds chicken wings
- Toasted sesame seeds for garnish

Directions:

1. Mix all ingredients except the sesame seeds.
2. Stir to coat the chicken wings.
3. Cook on low for 6 hours.
4. Garnish with sesame seeds.

Nutrition information: Calories per serving: 475; Carbohydrates: 3g; Protein: 31.8g; Fat: 21g; Sugar: 0g; Sodium: 274mg; Fiber: 0.9g

CHICKEN AND KALE TORTILLA STEW

Preparation Time: 55 Minutes

Serves: 6

Ingredients:

- 4 c. of kale, stems removed and chopped
- 1 tsp. cumin powder
- 6 c. chicken broth
- 2 tbsps. chili powder
- 2 large chicken breasts
- 1 tsp. paprika
- 1 can crushed tomatoes
- 2 tsps. garlic powder
- 1 can sweet corn
- ¼ c. lime juice, freshly squeezed
- ¼ c. Greek yogurt
- 1 can green chilies
- 2 tbsps. minced garlic

Directions:

1. Take all ingredients except the Greek yogurt in

the Crockpot.

2. Give a stir to mix all ingredients.

3. Cook on low for 5 hours.

4. Add the Greek yogurt and continue cooking on high for another hour.

Nutrition information: Calories per serving: 362; Carbohydrates: 10g; Protein: 25g; Fat: 10g; Sugar: 1.5g; Sodium: 159mg; Fiber: 6.3g

ITALIAN CHICKEN WITH ZUCCHINI NOODLES

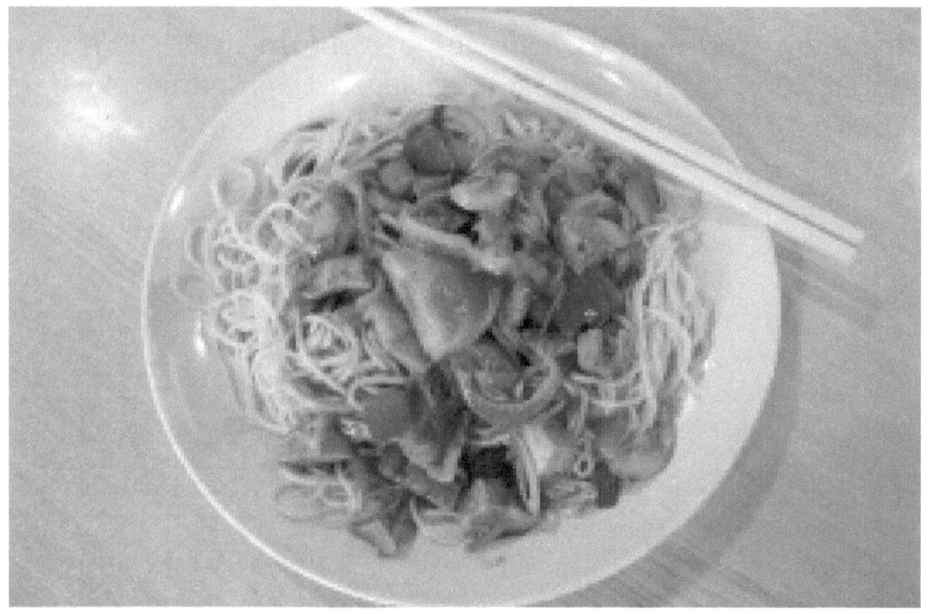

Preparation Time: 1 hour 10 Minutes

Serves: 6

Ingredients:

- ½ c. chicken broth
- 1 tsp. Italian seasoning
- 4 tsps. tomato paste
- 1-pound chicken breast

- 2 tomatoes, chopped
- 1 ½ c. asparagus
- 1 c. snap peas, halved
- Pepper and salt to taste
- 4 zucchini noodles, cut into noodle-like strips
- 1 c. commercial pesto
- Parmesan cheese for garnish
- Basil for garnish

Directions:

1. Take the chicken broth, Italian seasoning, tomato paste, chicken breasts, tomatoes, asparagus, and peas in the Crockpot. Give a swirl and season with pepper and salt to taste.

2. Close the lid and cook on low for 6 hours. Let it cool before assembling.

3. Assemble the noodles by placing the chicken mixture on top of the zucchini noodles. Add commercial pesto and garnish with parmesan cheese and basil leaves.

Nutrition information: Calories per serving: 429.7; Carbohydrates:6 g; Protein: 32g; Fat: 26g; Sugar:0.4 g; Sodium: mg; Fiber: 4.2g

CHAPTER 10:
APPETIZERS AND DESSERT

CROCKPOT KETO CHOCOLATE CAKE

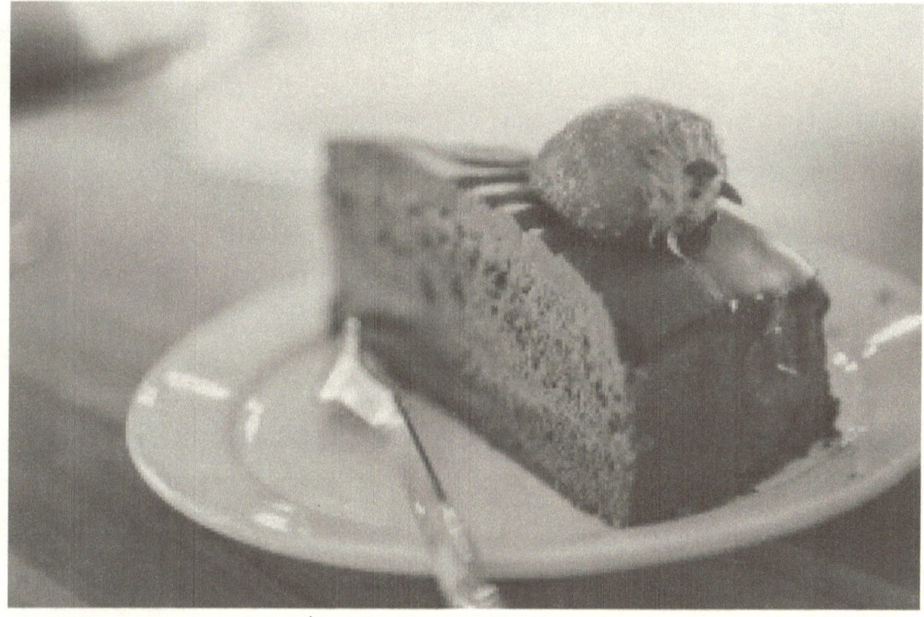

Preparation Time: 20 Minutes

Serves: 12

Ingredients:

- ¾ c. stevia sweetener
- 1 ½ c. almond flour
- ¼ tsp. baking powder
- ¼ c. protein powder, chocolate, or vanilla flavor

- 2/3 c. unsweetened cocoa powder
- ¼ tsp. salt
- ½ c. unsalted butter, melted
- 4 large eggs
- ¾ c. heavy cream
- 1 tsp. vanilla extract

Instructions:

1. Grease the ceramic insert of the Crockpot.
2. In a bowl, mix the sweetener, almond flour, protein powder, cocoa powder, salt, and baking powder.
3. Add the butter, eggs, cream, and vanilla extract.
4. Pour the batter in the Crockpot and cook on low for 3 hours.
5. Allow to cool before slicing.

Nutrition information: Calories per serving: 253; Carbohydrates: 5.1g; Protein: 17.3g; Fat: 29.5g; Sugar: 1.2g; Sodium: 361mg; Fiber: 2.4g

KETO CROCKPOT CHOCOLATE LAVA CAKE

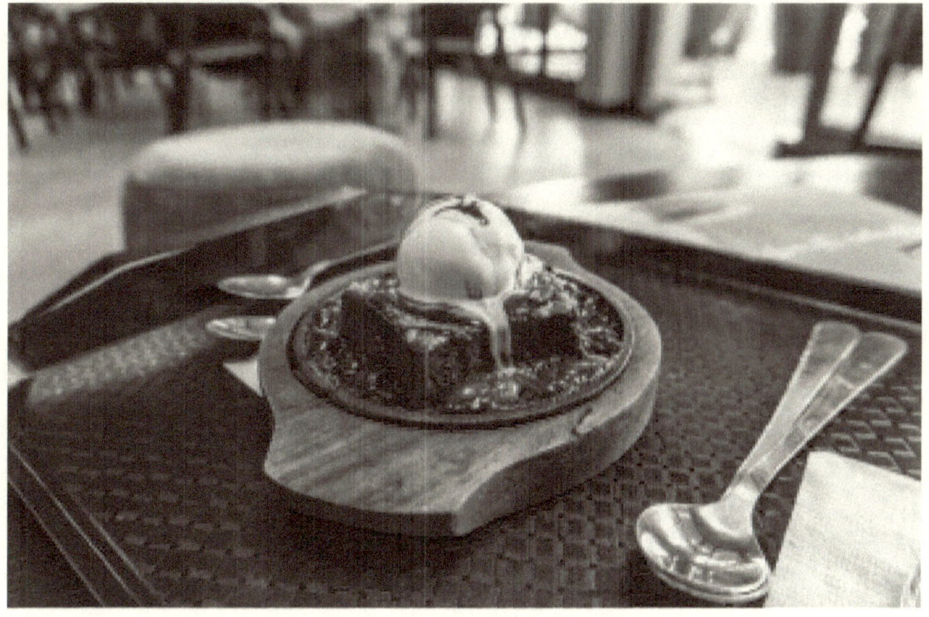

Preparation Time: 30 Minutes

Serves: 12

Ingredients:

- 1 ½ c. stevia sweetener, divided

- ½ c. almond flour

- 5 tbsps. unsweetened cocoa powder

- ½ tsp. salt

- 1 tsp. baking powder
- 3 whole eggs
- 3 egg yolks
- ½ c. butter, melted
- 1 tsp. vanilla extract
- 2 c. hot water
- 4 ounces sugar-free chocolate chips

Instructions:

1. Grease the inside of the Crockpot.
2. In a bowl, mix the stevia sweetener, almond flour, cocoa powder, salt, and baking powder.
3. In another bowl, mix the eggs, egg yolks, butter, and vanilla extract. Pour in the hot water.
4. Pour the wet ingredients to the dry ingredients and fold to create a batter.
5. Add the chocolate chips last
6. Pour into the greased Crockpot and cook on low for 3 hours.
7. Allow to cool before serving.

Nutrition information: Calories per serving: 157; Carbohydrates: 5.5g; Protein: 10.6g; Fat: 13g; Sugar:0.2 g; Sodium: 155mg; Fiber: 2.6g

LEMON CROCKPOT CAKE

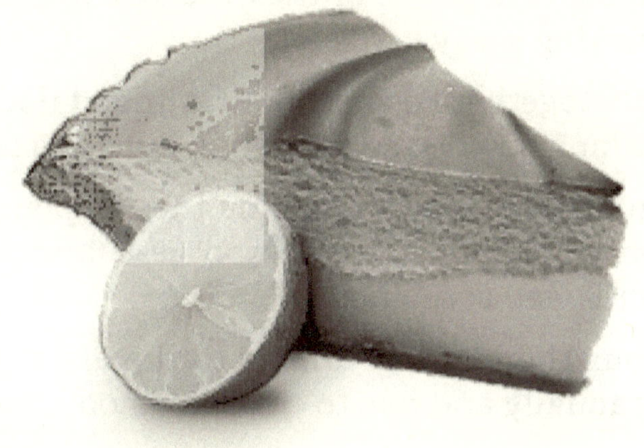

Preparation Time: 15 Minutes

Serves: 8

Ingredients:

- ½ c. coconut flour
- 1 ½ c. almond flour
- 3 tbsps. stevia sweetener
- 2 tsps. baking powder
- ½ tsp. xanthan gum
- ½ c. whipping cream
- ½ c. butter, melted
- 1 tbsp. juice, freshly squeezed

- Zest from one large lemon
- 2 eggs

Instructions:

1. Grease the inside of the Crockpot with butter or cooking spray.
2. Mix together coconut flour, almond flour, stevia, baking powder, and xanthan gum in a bowl.
3. In another bowl, combine the whipping cream, butter, lemon juice, lemon zest, and eggs. Mix until well combined.
4. Pour the wet ingredients to the dry ingredients gradually and fold to create a smooth batter.
5. Spread the batter in the Crockpot and cook on low for 3 hours or until a toothpick inserted in the middle comes out clean.

Nutrition information: Calories per serving: 350; Carbohydrates: 11.1g; Protein:17.6 g; Fat: 32.6g; Sugar: 0.9g; Sodium: 224mg; Fiber: 4.9g

KETO BASIC VANILLA CAKE IN A CROCKPOT

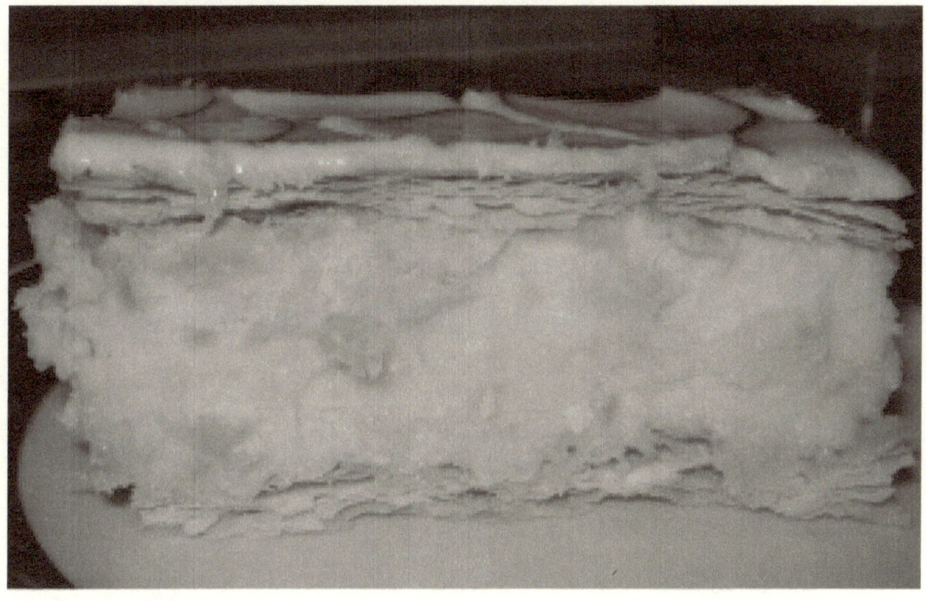

Preparation Time: 25 Minutes

Serves: 12

Ingredients:

- ¼ tsp. salt
- 1 ½ c. almond flour
- ¾ c. stevia sweetener
- 2/3 c. protein powder, vanilla powder

- ¾ c. heavy cream
- 2 tsps. baking powder
- 4 large eggs
- ½ c. unsalted butter, melted
- 1 tsp. vanilla extract

Instructions:

1. Grease the insert of the Crockpot with cooking spray.
2. In a bowl, mix the almond flour, sweetener, protein powder, salt, and baking powder.
3. In another bowl, combine the butter, heavy cream, eggs, and vanilla extract.
4. Pour the wet ingredients to the dry ingredients and fold to create a smooth batter.
5. Pour into the greased Crockpot.
6. Cook on low for 3 hours.
7. Let it cool before serving.

Nutrition information: Calories per serving: 162; Carbohydrates: 4.1g; Protein: 11.6g; Fat: 12.3g; Sugar: 2.3g; Sodium: 154mg; Fiber:0.5 g

MOCHA PUDDING CAKE

Preparation Time: 60 Minutes

Serves: 6

Ingredients:

- ¾ c. butter, cut into chunks
- 2 ounces unsweetened chocolate, chopped
- ½ c. heavy cream
- 2 tbsps. instant coffee
- 1 tsp. vanilla extract
- 1/3 c. almond flour
- 4 tbsps. cocoa powder, unsweetened
- 1/8 tsp. salt
- 5 large eggs
- 2/3 c. stevia sweetener

Instructions:

1. Grease the Crockpot pot with cooking spray or butter.

2. In a double boiler, melt the butter and unsweetened chocolate over medium heat. Once melted, remove from heat, and allow to cool.

3. In a small bowl, combine the heavy cream, coffee,

and vanilla extract.

4. In another bowl, combine the almond flour, cocoa powder, and salt.

5. Beat the eggs in a large bowl and add the stevia sweetener until slightly thickened or until it turns pale yellow.

6. To the egg mixture, pour in the melted chocolate. Whisk until combined. Add the flour mixture gradually while continuously whisking.

7. Pour in the coffee mixture last. Whisk until combined.

8. Pour the batter into the Crockpot.

9. Place a paper towel on top of the Crockpot before closing the lid.

10. Cook on low for 3 hours.

Nutrition information: Calories per serving: 414; Carbohydrates: 3.8g; Protein: 10.9g; Fat: 38.9g; Sugar: 13g; Sodium: 542mg; Fiber:0.9 g

CINNAMON BLONDIE PECAN BARS

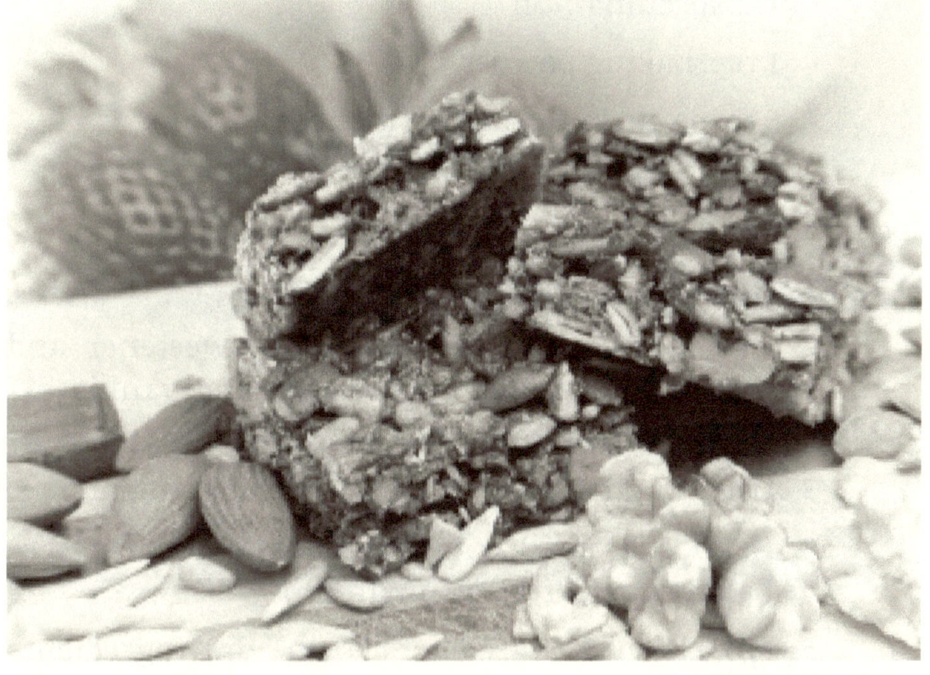

Preparation Time: 55 Minutes

Serves: 16

Ingredients:

- 1 c. stevia sweetener
- 1 c. pecans, chopped
- 3 large eggs

- ¼ c. heavy whipping cream
- 1 ½ c. almond flour
- 2 tsps. vanilla extract
- 2 tbsps. unsalted butter
- ¼ tsp. salt
- 1 tbsp. cinnamon
- 1 tsp. baking powder
- 6 tbsps. unsalted butter, melted

Instructions:

1. Grease the Crockpot with butter.
2. In a bowl, combine the stevia sweetener and melted butter. Add in the eggs and vanilla extract.
3. Use a hand mixer to combine the ingredients.
4. In another bowl, combine the almond flour, salt, baking powder, and cinnamon.
5. Mix the wet ingredients to the dry ingredients until combined.
6. Pour the dough in the Crockpot and press to form a dense bar.
7. Cook on low for 3 hours.
8. Meanwhile, mix the butter, whipping cream, and pecans in a saucepan. Allow to boil and reduce slightly.
9. Once the bars are cooked, pour over the pecan sauce.

Nutrition information: Calories per serving: 190.6; Carbohy-drates: 1.9g; Protein: 4.42g; Fat: 20.56g; Sugar: 0.5g; Sodium: 163mg; Fiber:0 g

Crockpot Dark Chocolate Cake

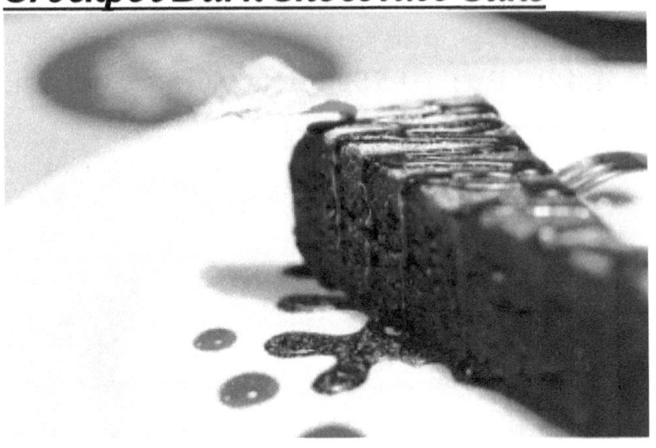

Preparation Time: 40 Minutes

Serves: 10

Ingredients:

- 1 c. almond flour
- ½ c. cocoa powder
- ½ c. stevia sweetener
- 3 tbsps. whey protein powder, unflavored
- 1 ½ tsps. baking powder
- ¼ tsp. salt
- 3 large eggs
- 2/3 c. unsweetened almond milk
- 6 tbsps. butter, melted
- ¾ tsp. vanilla extract
- 1/3 c. sugar-free chocolate chips

Instructions:

1. Grease the Crockpot with butter.

2. In a medium bowl, whisk the almond flour, cocoa powder, stevia powder, and whey protein. Add in the baking powder and salt.

3. In another bowl, combine the eggs, almond milk, butter, and vanilla extract.

4. Pour the wet ingredients to the dry ingredients and whisk until the batter is smooth.

5. Add the chocolate chips last.

6. Pour the batter in the Crockpot and bake on low for 3 hours.

Nutrition information: Calories per serving: 205; Carbohydrates:8.42 g; Protein: 7.37g; Fat: 16.79g; Sugar: 0.3g; Sodium: 230mg; Fiber: 4.1g

EASY CROCKPOT CHEESECAKE

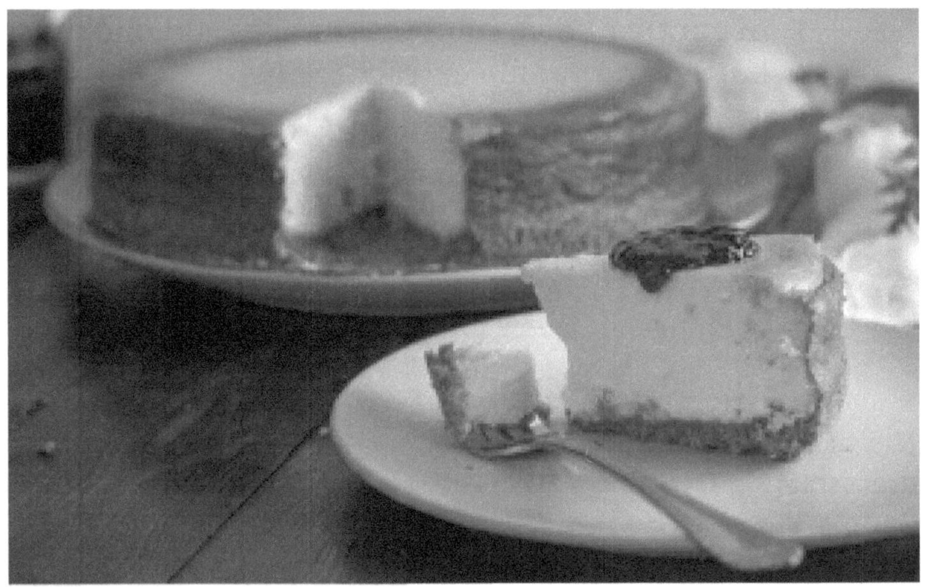

Preparation Time: 35 Minutes

Serves: 6

Ingredients:

- 3 8-ounce cream cheese, room temperature
- 1 c. stevia sweetener
- 3 eggs
- ½ tbsp. vanilla extract

Instructions:

1. Grease the Crockpot with butter.
2. In a mixing bowl, mix the cream cheese and stevia sweetener.
3. Use a hand mixer to mix everything.
4. Add the eggs and vanilla extract.
5. Pour the mixture into the Crockpot and cook on low for 3 hours.

Nutrition information: Calories per serving: 264; Carbohydrates:3g; Protein: 9.1g; Fat: 15.8g; Sugar: 2.6g; Sodium: 157mg; Fiber: 0g

CONCLUSION

Thank you again for owning this book!

I hope this book was able to help you understand the keto diet as well as the keto slow cooker recipes.

By now, I am confident that you know the essentials of the keto diet for your pantry and kitchen. You know how to shop and the right containers to store your food for the week.

We did not stop there; we looked at the importance of macros for keto meal planning and got insights on how to calculate macros and why we should.

The next step is for you to take the insights and tips from this book and ingratiate them into your keto plan. The benefits are numerous, and the joy you will get from the information and the recipes in this book is invaluable.

Thank you, and good luck!